Ṛ … ā

An… …cience behind
Menstrual Practices

SINU JOSEPH

notionpress
.com

INDIA • SINGAPORE • MALAYSIA

Notion Press

No.8, 3rd Cross Street,
CIT Colony, Mylapore,
Chennai, Tamil Nadu – 600004

First Published by Notion Press 2020

ISBN 978-1-64919-866-2

To the Master who pointed me in the direction in which to seek, and transformed my ability to perceive, simply by placing his hands on my head,

I remain eternally grateful.

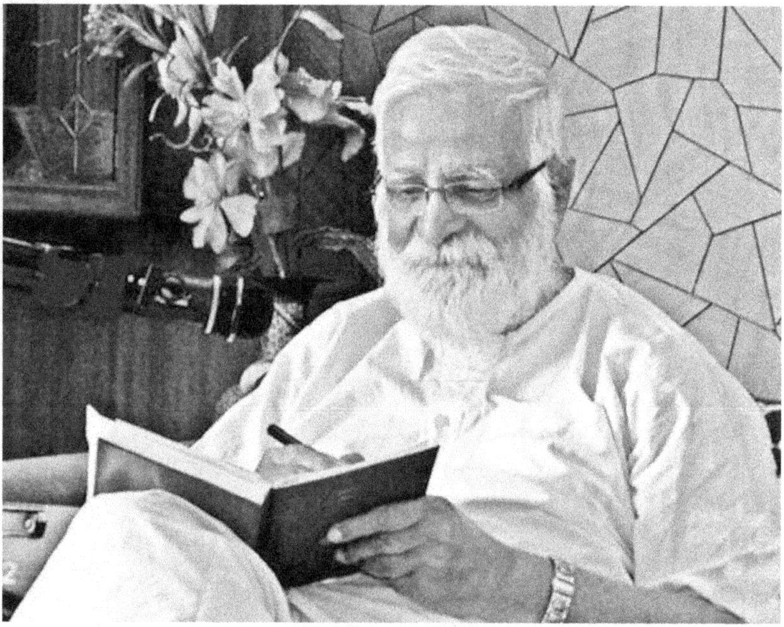

Pūjya Śrī Amritānanda Nātha Saraswati

(Dr. Nishtala Prahlada Sastry)

Founder of Devīpuram

26th September 1934 - 10th October 2015

"What is pure, we do not touch. And what we do not touch, we call it a taboo. She (a menstruating woman) was so pure, that she was worshipped as a Goddess. The reason for not having a woman go into a temple is precisely this. She is a living Goddess at that time."[1]

– Pūjya Śrī Amritānanda Nātha Saraswati

1 Excerpts from my conversation with Guruji in 2015 at his residence in Vishakhapatnam, Andhra Pradesh, India. Details are provided in Chapter 8 of this book.

Photo credit: William Thomas

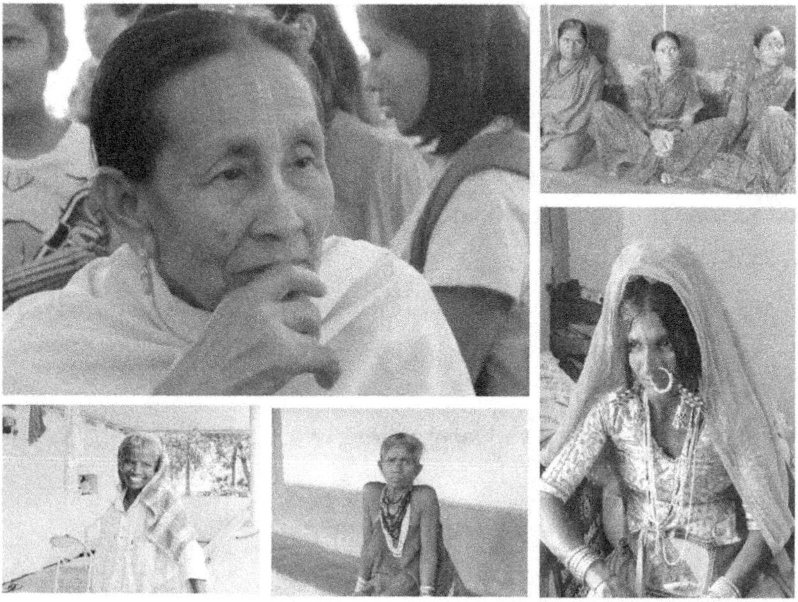

Image credit: Taken by the author during her interactions with women from rural India.

To,

The Grandmothers of Rural India

The keepers of our culture and tradition;

Through their faith, we heal;

Through their wisdom, we learn;

Through their discipline, we return

To our roots.

Oh, what would we, the ignorant modern women,
do without them!

Special Dedication

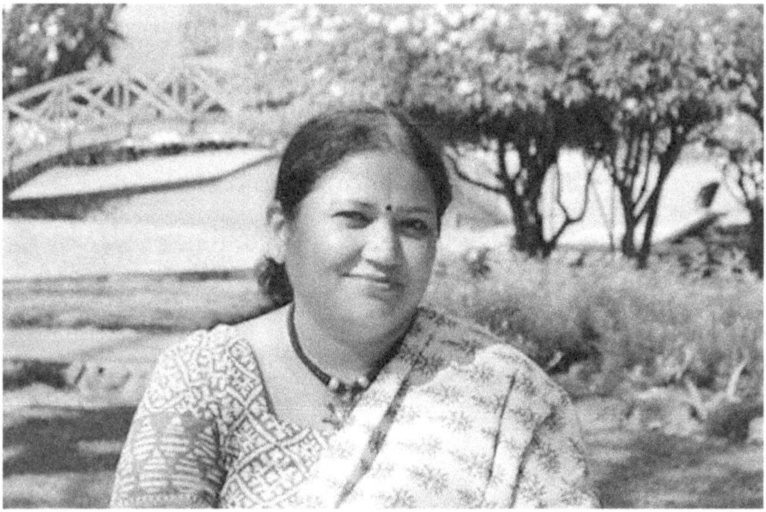

Smt. Vyjayanthi Krishnamurthy

June 25, 1962 – October 03, 2019

I have been greatly blessed to have had you as a companion and guide in my work for nearly ten years. We started this journey together and you have been with me every step of the way. This book is the culmination of our work together. It is yours as much as it is mine.

Contents

About the Title 13

Sanskrit Pronunciation Guide 15

Foreword 17

Preface 29

Acknowledgments 37

PART I : Menstruation in Science

Introduction to Part I: What is Ancient Science? 43

Chapter 1: Menarche: The Need for Celebration 69

Chapter 2: Decoding Menstrual Practices through Āyurved 105

Chapter 3: Menstrual Blood: Impure or Highly Pure? 134

Chapter 4: Menstrual Seclusion: What Women Need 141

Chapter 5: Sports and Menstruation: Why It Doesn't Have to Be Painful 150

Chapter 6: Celestial Influence on Menstrual Cycles 174

Chapter 7: Gifts of the Menstrual Cycle 204

PART II: Menstruation in Religion

Introduction to Part II: Hinduism as a Religion 221

Chapter 8: How Do Hindu Temples Impact Menstruation? 235

Chapter 9: Chengannur Bhagavathy: The Temple that Aligns Menstrual Cycles 262

Chapter 10: Mantras and Their Effect on Menstrual Cycles 272

Chapter 11: Kāmākhya: Where Menstruation Meets Spirituality 285

Chapter 12: The Myth of Menstruation as a Result of Indrā's Sin 313

Chapter 13: Menstrual Practices in Christianity and Islam 322

Notes

1. Darśana 331
2. Dhātu 353
3. Pañcamahābhūta 357
4. Sub types of Doṣa 360
5. Ṣat Rasa – The Six Tastes 365
6. Ṣat Cakra – The Six Cakras 372

Index 379

About the Title

Ṛtu (pronounced as ruthu) is one of the words in Sanskrit for menstruation. Vidyā means knowledge. Ṛtu Vidyā is the author's attempt to bring together various Indian knowledge systems that provide information about the science of menstruation, which is relevant even to this day.

Image credit:

The painting on the cover page is an original work by artist Ms. Manisha Raju from Chennai, India.

Sanskrit Pronunciation Guide

In this book, I have used the International Alphabet of Sanskrit Transliteration (IAST) for words and names that were originally in Sanskrit (henceforth written as Saṃskṛtam), even though some of the words like Yoga, Chakra, or Ayurveda might have become part of the English language in recent times. Given that this book is an attempt to capture the original meaning of various practices around menstruation, I felt that it is imperative to also include the original Saṃskṛtam words the way in which they were meant to be pronounced, as a reminder to seek the source while decoding Indian knowledge systems. The pronunciations as per IAST are given below.

a	u in but	ḍa	d in dust
ā	a in star	ḍha	dh in adhere
i	i in bit	ṇa	n in under
ī	ee in teeth	ta	t in thumb
u	u in put	tha	aspirated ta
ū	oo in mood	da	th in the
ṛ	r in rough	dha	aspirated da
ṛ¯	longer ṛ	na	n in not
e	a in mane	pa	p in spill
o	o in go	pha	p in pill
ō	o in odor	ba	b in bill
ai	combination of a and i	bha	aspirated b
au	combination of a and u	ma	m in mail
ka	k in skill	ya	y in yellow
kh	kh in khakhi	ra	r in run
ga	g in gun	la	l in light
gha	gh in Ghana	va	v in vase
ṅa	ng in lung	śa	s in shine
ca	c in inch	ṣa	s in push
cha	c in church	sa	s in see
ja	j in jug	ha	voiced h
jha	j in Jhansi	aṃ	sum
ña	n in lunch	aḥ	aha
ṭa	t in time	jña	gnya
ṭha	th in anthill	hma, hna	mha, nha

FOREWORD

In Ṛtu Vidyā, Sinu Joseph has gifted us a remarkably insightful book describing her own journey of understanding menstrual phenomena, a core expression of being a female human. The author does this by connecting stories of many women across India and merging her own story with theirs. Ṛtu Vidyā then unfolds these connections by describing them through the lens of practices of Indian traditions based on the Vedas, including Āyurved, Jyotiṣa, Mantra and Tantra Śāstra.

Ṛtu Vidyā follows the author's book 'Women and Sabarimala' published in 2019 (which made it to Amazon's best seller lists in Hinduism category for long periods of time), using the lens of Veda based Śāstra behind the architecture of Devasthanās to describe the impact of Sabarimala on women.

For me, this book represents one of the first signals of an emerging renaissance at the lokavyāvahārika level, a rebirth of a vibrant Indian culture which connects, enlivens and enables flourishing of all that makes up India – humans, animals, plants, forests, rivers, mountains. In our Śrutis, Smritis and Purāṇa all of the cosmos and all manifestations on Earth are described as having sentience. Modernity has shorn us from this core insight. Modernity considers humans as central and the only sentient in the cosmos, while rendering everything else insentient. The result is apparent in the ecocide, the deadly destruction of our ecology, all around us – because specifically modern humans are considered defacto superior to non-modern humans and of course to the rest of cosmos. This book shows us how we can begin to recover: by beginning to make sense of the cultural practices that evolved over millennia based on the core insights about the cosmos and the nature of humans. It does so by taking up the quintessential phenomena of menstruation that not only is evocative of the female human manifestation, but also central to sustenance of the human species. In the process of doing so, it brings to the fore how the modern lens has distorted cultural practices which it considers foreign to it.

It is important to understand the intellectual roots of the distortion of non-modern cultural practices that the modern lens gives rise to. Such distortion has driven cultural destruction of multiple human cultures around the world. The homogenization of human culture has led to loss of diversity, which parallels the loss of diversity we notice in our forests, our gardens and our ways of living. The success of the European Enlightenment in resolving Europe's problem of incessant religious and civil war from the 13th to 15th centuries and to empower it with the apparent ability to dominate nature (at least in the relatively short term of a few hundred years) led to Europe's drive to colonize the world. And with it came an intellectual hubris best captured by Hegel's (1770-1831) view as I paraphrased in my essay[2]:

---

2 https://www.amazon.com/OUTSIDER-DECONSTRUCTING-EUROPEAN-ENLIGHTENMENT-Death-ebook/dp/B07RHVRV7V

> European horizon transcended all Asian horizons. Asian thought was comprehensible and interpretable within European thought but not vice versa. The question of an adequate standpoint for the evaluation and comparison of different cultural traditions had, according to Hegel, been decided by the course of history itself, and it had been decided in favour of Europe. European thought, therefore, had to provide the context and the categories for the exploration of all traditions of thought.[3]

As you begin reading this book there will be a number of questions that will arise. You will be reading this in English. So implicitly you will be using the western lens. Those questions will begin to distort what the author is conveying here for quite a few of you who are not practitioners of Indian traditions as well. It is to those who are navigating modernity while being practitioners of Indian traditions that this book is most likely to begin making sense. Perhaps you, dear reader, is one such. Perhaps it will help you to begin recovering the lens that your ancestors developed over millennia of observation and experimenting of how to live a balanced and fulfilling life. And hopefully you may begin to adapt those views into your cultural way of life and thus enable more and more people around you to flourish.

And I do not mean that as an empty flourish. The female human plays a most critical role in the flourishing of human manifestation. Yet, modernity completely subsumes woman's

---

3 Pp 32 Halbfass, Wilhelm, India International Centre Quarterly Vol. 16, No. 2 (SUMMER 1989), pp. 29-44 https://www.jstor.org/stable/23002139?seq=1

role as the creatrix and mother, by putting gross material flourishing on the pedestal. All metrics which govern our modern way of life, whether in terms of time or effort (think productivity, efficiency, effectiveness etc.) makes us focus on exploitation of what modernity deems to be resources for material production and consumption. Menstruation plays a central role in a woman's life cycle. The technology to manage and to suppress menstrual cycles so that women's bodies are free to shift the focus on increasing material productivity (marketed as economic freedom) is a central toxic hallmark of modernity. And we are all participants in sustaining these modern processes. Many of us may be actively subverting any opposition to modernity (and how it shapes women, whether through the stance of 'conservative' modernity or 'progressive' modernity) that may arise from competing cultural paradigms that describe creative roles women play in human flourishing. Ṛtu Vidyā offers a competing vision of humans and women to the one offered up by the modern paradigm. As the book gets traction and attention, it is likely to attract vehement opposition from many moderns who see freedom only in narrow economic terms and in effect as the unbounded opportunity to bond ourselves to the treadmill of ever increasing material efficiency demanded as sacrifice at the altar of Capital.

Let me explore what some of the thrusts of the modern opposition may be, which perhaps would be led directly or indirectly by academics and researchers, both in western and Indian academia. This is important for you, dear reader, to understand. So that you read the book keeping in mind that it uses a different lens than the one which is ubiquitous in the dominant global material economic framework, to which we are all bound to in this era of techno-financial globalization.

Ṛtu Vidyā describes menstruation using two broad frameworks: through science and through religion. The science it describes is based on knowledge gained through observation of evidence over a long period of time applied to a framework of what is human (the pañca kośa, the five sheaths, for example) and how the human is integral with and connected to the cosmos (the principle that drives the macro, the cosmos, is the principle that drives the smallest part of the human cell). It is thus both evidence based and theory based. The evidence is not top down laboratory based that the West would demand as a way of demonizing democratic science. It is a democratic science of the people sharing evidence and over period of time coming up with rules, heuristics. This is a process that has been going on over many millennia. Modern science, especially in the English speaking world, has a specific origin. In the Royal Society chartered by King Charles II of England in 1660. From then onwards, all science had to pass through a top down peer review, with peers being appointed by the Crown. Science came under the domain of authority. No investigation or its results were to be considered scientific unless it was accepted and published in the Philosophical Transactions of the Royal Society which made its first appearance in print in 1665 (this journal is now the oldest scientific journal in continuous publication in the world and established the concepts of scientific priority and peer review[4]). This is the structure of modern science, with its roots a little over 300 years deep and centered in Europe, and the consequent modern scientific knowledge and the technology, including financial technology that now dominates the globe. Western academia and western influenced Indian

4 https://royalsociety.org/about-us/history/

academia and scientists are missionaries of this system of authority of controlled top down knowledge. Moderns in general, and its academics and researchers in particular, will use the lens of modern science when they read Ṛtu Vidyā and will see and describe a distorted view.

The framework of religion that Ṛtu Vidyā employs to describe menstruation is the Hindu framework. From the modern perspective this approach is doomed from the beginning. The strategy of intellectual colonizing by Europe had the following broad steps: Christian missionaries came in and 'studied' texts (written and oral) of a culture and discerned a religion. In collaboration with intellectuals in their home countries they described and declared a religion that these backward peoples follow. They then compared and contrasted this new religion, which they had discovered and described, with the Bible and declared the newly discovered religion to be false. Declaring a religion false is the pre-set goal of missionaries, thus valorizing their one and only true religion. Thus, only Christianity (while acknowledging its Judaic roots) is the one true religion. Justice and love can only flow from this one true religion. False religions are deemed to be oppressive and cruel. Once such comparative template was established, it was applied to every aspect of cultural life in India, deeming all of it as backward, childish, superstitious, oppressive and cruel. It was used to break down the cultural-meaning-structure, the linkages and guidelines that people used to go about in this world. A broken culture is fertile ground for intellectual colonization by the modern paradigm. And the moderns of the West as of now see it as an unfinished project. This is Jurgen Habermas, a much respected German philosopher (1929 -) continuing the lineage of Hegel about the supremacy of the West over the rest:

> "Universalistic egalitarianism," he stated in a 2002 interview, "is the direct legacy of the Judaic ethic of justice and the Christian ethic of love... Up to this very day there is no alternative to it." Drawing a dubious contrast between the two monotheistic religions, Habermas articulated what would become the core of his intellectual program. The West's Judeo-Christian heritage was not a passing phase in the emergence of modern thought and politics, but contributed—and perhaps still contributes—its essential core.[5]

The message is clear. The foundation of rational discourse of modern science to move society towards justice and love is based on Judeo-Christian heritage of the West. That is the true religion. Any attempt to bring in what the Western intellectual deems as a false religion to sustain pre-modern cultural paradigms will be seen as part of the unfinished project of modernizing the world. To be either converted or extinguished.

Such intellectual colonization has made deep roots in India. Those of us who consider ourselves as modern in India wait for innovation to trickle down from the West, which we then mimic. That mimicry defines much of the English-speaking world of India. Into this reality on the ground comes Ṛtu Vidyā. The book openly and confidently uses the Hindu framework to describe how Indian women manage their menstrual health and reality of its Devashthānas and its related practices.

As the book begins to get substantial traction among Indian readers, aggressive critique may be expected of both the book

---

5 http://bostonreview.net/philosophy-religion/brandon-bloch-unfinished-project-enlightenment?utm_source=pocket-newtab

and the author, as being pre-modern, anti-women's liberation, anti-science, superstitious, oppressive etc. Such aggressive critique will be a sign that what Ṛtu Vidyā is saying is seen as a threat to the unfinished project of the global homogenization mission of modern science. One hopes that such aggressive critique would be seen as a positive challenge to the Indian readers of the book to go deeper into their cultural practices, and also to become even more adept at navigating and succeeding in the modern materialist world. While at the same time begin to refashion the way we go about in the world, especially in what we produce and consume, so that more and more have the opportunity to build capacity to practice Mokṣa Śāstra at earlier stages in their life cycle.

It is perhaps this refashioning in mind that Ṛtu Vidyā consciously uses Sanskrit terms (and yes, one of the aggressive critiques from the progressive moderns will be that all of Sanskrit is oppressive), without translating them into English. Let me explain. Language with its vocabulary and grammar are used by a culture to create networks (or webs) of meanings. The web of meanings we construct each time we write or speak a sentence is transmitted and communicated to those around us. The web of meanings creates a visualization in the listener/ reader and this visualization becomes the 'real' world through which we interact and transact with each other. It's the way we go about in the world and do business. These webs of meanings interact in complex ways. Let's call it the memetic complex.[6] The memetic complexes, which carry powerful meanings

6 A term I have used quite often in my essay https://www.amazon.com/OUTSIDER-DECONSTRUCTING-EUROPEAN-ENLIGHTENMENT-Death-ebook/dp/B07RHVRV7V

upon which narratives explaining how to go about in the world, (build institutions and contracts between individuals, assigning roles and thus creating hierarchies) are constructed, are closely guarded by the keepers of the lexicon, vocabulary and grammar. The Oxford Dictionary, for example, is considered the central depository of meanings in the English language. The constructors of narratives are influential academics (e.g. faculty at Harvard University), authors (popular science authors such as Stewart Brand[7]) and journalists (e.g. those employed by New York Times). There may be many readers who complain that the Sanskrit words used in Ṛtu Vidyā do not make sense to them and therefore they cannot appreciate the book. They will ask for simple translation into English. The key Sanskrit words that have been retained in Ṛtu Vidyā (e.g. Prāṇa Pratiṣṭha) are part of a meaning network. They are not standalone. If that word is translated into a single word in English (in this case consecration), two things happen: one, the meaning network signaled by the word Prāṇa Pratiṣṭha is lost. The word is shorn from the entire meaning network and visualization in the Indian cultural ecosystem that evokes in the reader who is immersed in the culture. In the translation, if the word consecration is used, it will evoke a meaning network that is integral to Western Christianity and the cultural ethos of Europe. So through such translation of key words that define the interface between lokavyāvāhāra and Mokṣa Śāstra, the core of Indian culture is obfuscated. The process of decolonizing requires recovery of this core interface of meaning networks in Indian culture. Ṛtu Vidyā makes a beginning in this direction, by retaining use of

7 https://www.newyorker.com/news/letter-from-silicon-valley/the-complicated-legacy-of-stewart-brands-whole-earth-catalog

key Sanskrit words and describing the meaning network that they support, with examples to assist readers to understand.

Since you have reached here in reading this rather long and dense foreword, I take it that you are a serious reader. I would like to suggest a way to read this book using the process suggested in our traditions for engaging with Mokṣa Śāstra: Śravaṇaṃ, Mananam, Nididhyāsanam. This book shows how the lok vyavahāra phenomena of women managing menstruation is linked to the interface with Mokṣa Śāstra, through the Darśanas and through Āgama Śāstra. It is therefore best appreciated by adopting the 3-step process. One way of doing so in the 21st century may be to come together in small study groups of 3 to 5 through weekly online meetings. Take up a few pages of reading from the book at each of the study group meetings. That is Śravaṇaṃ (listening or reading). After reading for about 15 minutes or so, reflect on the reading and share your sense of the reading. For example, if the reading is about a visit to a Devasthanā, you may share your experience of a similar visit. Or share questions that came to mind when you went through the reading. Have a non-judgmental discussion. That is Mananam. Each weekly study group session of a total of 40 minutes may suffice. The third part of the process, Nididhyāsanam, paying attention to how you can make some learning from the study group session to begin changing how you view certain aspects of the world. And as that happens, there begins emerging a change to some of the things you do and how you do it. Once you experience this process, beginning to make changes in you, it may become so much easier for you to take up a Mokṣa Śāstra text such as the Bhagavad Gītā and go through a similar process. You may be surprised by the cognitive shifts that the process brings to you when you are in a positively guided study group. I hope the author sets up a way to train study group facilitators and setting up of such groups, after this book is published. The gender composition of such study groups and who should lead them is something that may need to be designed after thinking things through.

I do hope you, dear reader, will take time to closely read Ṛtu Vidyā. I hope it begins to enable you to use the lens from your own culture to view the world. A lens that has been latent and clouded over, and perhaps denigrated, by the dominant techno-financial paradigm.

– Jayant Kalawar

New Jersey, USA

PREFACE

Every once in a while, I receive a request from menstrual researchers and activists asking me to pinpoint them to ancient texts which explain why Indian women follow certain practices such as avoiding specific types of food, cooking, touching others, or entering Hindu temples during menstruation. How I wish such information readily existed, as it would have spared me the difficult task of penning this book!

India's ancient texts have long lists of to-dos and not-to-dos prescribed for menstruating women, but rarely do they explain the reason behind this menstrual regime. That information is sacred and not revealed easily. To the one with faith, the questions never arise. To the one without faith, the answers must be earned, often through long and arduous journeys, both within and without.

The last five years of my decade-long work on menstruation have been spent on a journey traversing India and delving deep into India's indigenous sciences to piece together the varied information available on this topic. Although I read and re-read ancient texts and documents pertaining to this subject, my real understanding began only when I met and interacted with wise men and women from India. And most of all, when I myself experienced how cultural practices around menstruation, often dismissed as menstrual taboos, can help to prevent menstrual disorders.

There is a reason why such a book to decode the multitude of cultural practices around menstruation in India, through a scientific lens, has not happened before. Firstly, India's traditional knowledge systems, which form the basis of these practices, have been sidelined as 'alternate systems', and the subtle sciences that they represent have not been fully acknowledged in the modern scientific community. Secondly, to fully grasp even the simplest cultural practice, there is a need to study diverse topics, from Āyurved to Āgama Śāstra, all of which would be unfamiliar to those who have only dealt with Western sciences. And thirdly, unless this knowledge is clubbed with the experience of menstruation itself, the chances of erroneously interpreting cultural practices are high, as we see in articles and books on menstruation authored by male writers, regardless of good intention. There are, of course, exceptions to the rule. In the course of my own study, some of my greatest teachers have been men who, in their own lives, have gone beyond stereotypical definitions of gender and have been able to experience the feminine in profound ways.

In the chapters of this book, readers will find explanations of many of the cultural practices around menstruation that are currently followed by women in India.

The book is divided into two parts. In the first part of this book, each chapter delves into a different cultural practice, such as the celebration of menarche, the menstrual regime prescribed in ancient Āyurved texts, menstrual seclusion practices, and the notion of menstrual impurity. There is an exclusive chapter for sportswomen to understand their body through Āyurved, given that there is so little information for women in the menstrual age to go along with the natural rhythm of their menstrual cycle and yet be able to perform well in a physically demanding career.

In addition to these, there are some interesting facts about menstruation that have rarely, if at all, been spoken or written to date, such as the celestial influence on the female menstrual cycle and how women's cycles can be predicted through certain sciences. Part 1 of the book ends with the idea of why the menstrual cycle, as understood in ancient India, is a gift to womenkind and how it gives women an opportunity to tap into their unique cyclic patterns for enhanced productivity in work and life in general.

But this book is not just about decoding the science behind cultural practices around menstruation. It is also about inculcating a holistic understanding of menstruation as envisaged in the ancient texts of the Hindus. What did our ancestors know about menstruation that made them at once revere and fear menstruating women? The answer to this question is covered in the chapters of the second part of this book, where we delve into menstrual practices with respect to religion and spirituality. Many have questioned the seeming contradiction of menstruating women being restricted from entering Hindu temples or reciting certain mantras on the one hand and, on the other hand, celebrating the menstruation of Devī in temples like Kāmākhya. An attempt has been made to reconcile this seemingly contradictory perspective in the second part of this book.

The testimony and real experiences of women who have broken the rule and visited temples during menstruation are among the most important additions to this work. There is also a chapter that decodes, and if I may say, sets right, the well-known Hindu mythology of menstruation being a result of women incurring the sin of Indrā's crime of killing a brāhmaṇa. The second part of the book ends with a chapter that gives a peek into menstrual practices in Christianity and Islam, while explaining the absence of such practices in the Sikh religion.

As part of writing this book, I have enjoyed the study of various Indian knowledge systems, including the Ṣaḍ-Darśana, Āyurved, Tantra, Cakra, Yōg, Āgama Śāstra, Jyotiṣa Śāstra, and several sub-texts from these categories. Wherever possible, explanations from modern science and research have been studied and added to make it familiar and easier for readers to comprehend. The reason for studying such diverse topics was to understand the fundamental principles governing the idea behind the instructions in these texts, to go back to the basics of what these texts are meant to reveal, and to understand how the practices prescribed impact the human system, especially with respect to women's health.

This exercise has made me realize that in order to understand menstrual practices, it is a must to know the governing principles of multiple indigenous sciences because they are interconnected. Even to dismiss these practices as superstition or taboo, one needs to spend at least a few years learning the various sciences, from the knowledge of which such practices emerged. With so much 'homework' required, it is not difficult to imagine why there is a greater tendency to dismiss these practices as superstition or religious taboo, especially by those who are unfamiliar with Indian science, philosophy, and culture.

Having said that, this book would not have been complete with only a secondary study of the sciences and without the actual physical experience, and in the process gathering longitudinal evidence from many women, of how cultural practices prescribed during menstruation impact menstrual health. Just as modern scientific experiments create suitable 'lab conditions' to be able to test the hypothesis without external interference, in the case of experiencing the impact of menstrual practices too, such conditions need to be met internally. Therefore, I worked to bring my physical body to a state of good health, in order to rule out disturbances in the menstrual cycle owing to existing health issues. It was also important to bring the body and mind to a stable state through practices of yōg, prāṇāyāma, and meditation so that I could experience subtle changes during menstruation; this lies at the core of directly experiencing the effect of cultural practices during menstruation.

This book is also the result of rigorous groundwork over a period of ten years with my team, which included interactions with thousands of adolescent girls and women across the Indian states of Karnataka, Tamil Nadu, Andhra Pradesh, Kerala, Jharkhand, Bihar, Assam, Nagaland, Manipur, and Mizoram to get a first-hand perspective of cultural practices around menstruation which are followed to this day. Therefore, the practices chosen to be explained in this book have been arrived upon based on the current relevance and importance to Indian women.

To understand the impact of Hindu temples on menstrual cycles, temples such as the Bhagavathi temple in Chengannur (Kerala), the Valliyamkavu Devī temple in Mundakkayam

(Kerala), Umānanda temple and Kāmākhya temple in Guwahati (Assam), and five Sastha temples associated with Sabarimala in Tamil Nadu and Kerala were visited and are part of the study. Details pertaining to the restrictions on the entry of women in the menstrual age in Sabarimala were initially part of this work but were later published as a separate book titled Women and Sabarimala: The Science behind Restrictions, which was released in November 2019.

There has been a time in India when one did not have to explain rituals or religious practices. Our ancestors had a strong sense of unshakable devotion (bhakti), to not need a scientific explanation. This led them to have experiences that had the same effect as a scientific understanding. So, it was not uncommon that every time I interacted with genuinely religious people, in search of scientific answers, their question to me would always be 'but why do you want to know all that... just have bhakti.' So, why do we need to know all this through a scientific lens?

The influence of menstrual activists, both within and outside the country, who are unfamiliar with local traditions and culture, has done more harm than good. Their interference has, at times, resulted in governments making policies to enforce a change in traditional menstrual practices. A case in point is the government of Nepal introducing a law that criminalizes menstrual seclusion practices called chaupadi. While the law was unable to enforce an end to the practice, it did make practitioners go underground, further risking the safety of menstruating women. Another example is the case of the Sabarimala temple in Kerala that was forced by the Supreme Court of India in 2018 to remove its restriction on entry of women of menstruating age, following a petition backed by activists, leading to a massive uproar among devotees, both men and women.

At times, westerners have seen menstruation as a great opportunity for fame, often obtained by belittling cultural practices that are different from their own. An example of that is the documentary 'Period. End of Sentence', which shockingly won an Oscar award in 2019 for showcasing India as a country of people who disrespect menstruation and are blinded by menstrual taboos. With absolutely no knowledge of the culture they seek to condemn, and no effort to learn about native knowledge systems, such people somehow assume the authority to impose their limited thinking on the rest. Thus far, the voices commonly heard are of those who are backed by large organizations putting them on popular platforms to create a socially engineered narrative. This needs to change.

During the course of my study, I came across many women who never once felt that the cultural practices around menstruation have a negative connotation and chose to follow these practices with joy. I feel privileged to have learned from these wise women and their experiences. In some of the chapters in this book, you will find their version of the story.

Who is this book for?

This book is foremost for those women of India who have questioned the cultural practices around menstruation, at times being genuinely curious and at times by being rebellious.

This book is also for those who have difficulty in coming to terms with menstruation as a positive occurrence and assume that India has a cultural stigma around the subject.

This book is for the activist who is on a mission to 'empower' the women of India by asking her to forsake the cultural practices around menstruation.

This book is for the men who, in spite of good intentions, often speak on women's behalf without a clue about our body and our menstrual experience.

This book is for menstrual researchers, who will find several unexplored areas of research on menstrual health that can change the way we perceive menstruation.

This book is for the decision-makers who feel pressurized to go with the popular voice and lack the time and resources for a detailed study on such a subject.

Most readers will agree that books about women, written by women, through a feminine (not feminist) perspective, are rare. That such work will answer many, if not all, of the readers' questions on this subject is my sincere hope. That this book will encourage readers, especially women across the globe, to start their own journey of learning, surpassing and, wherever necessary, correcting what is presented here, through the lens of the native science of their motherland, is my deep desire. That, through this book, a fresh and meaningful scientific narrative on menstruation will emerge, that is not limited to Western scientific perspectives, will be a purpose met.

ACKNOWLEDGMENTS

First and foremost, I thank Pūjya Śrī Amritānanda Nātha Saraswathi, the founder of the Devīpuram temple in Andhra Pradesh. He was the first person who turned my thinking on this subject and pointed me in the right direction to seek answers.

I sincerely thank Śrī Jayant Kalawar, who took the time and trouble to review this book and offer valuable suggestions, without which this book would not be what it is. He is an exponent in Advaita Vedānta, Yōg Sūtras, Śrī Vidyā, Systems Thinking, Antifragile Strategies, and a Life Coach. He is the one I turned to when something unusual happened that I could not decode—like the time when my menstrual cycle shifted by 13 days, following a visit to a particular temple. With his knowledge of ancient Indian sciences, he always took my journey a step forward.

I am immensely grateful to Dr. Ramya Bhat, an Āyurved physician, who helped me understand Āyurved in a more practical manner, through my own body's experiences. She is the one who lent me her medical textbooks on Āyurved and was thoughtful enough to dog-ear the pages that I must read! Through her treatment, I have witnessed many young women recover from severe menstrual disorders, including gynecologist-recommended surgical interventions.

Interactions with her made me realize how much good Āyurved's wisdom can do for women.

I am grateful to Dr. Jayashree Nataraj, for reviewing the chapters pertaining to Āyurved and for her valuable suggestions and additions to this work. As an Āyurved physician and academician, her inputs to the book have been immensely helpful. I also thank Shri Mahesh Vaidya and Smt. Padmakshi Vaidya, for supporting this work and connecting me to Dr. Jayashree Nataraj.

I sincerely thank Smt. Annapoorna Bhat, whose insights and knowledge of the ancient science of Indian astrology has helped me see menstruation in a whole new light. I am also grateful to her for the careful review of the chapter titled 'Celestial Influence on Menstrual Cycles', which could not have been completed without her support.

I thank Bhaskar, whose knowledge has helped me immensely in gaining a holistic perspective on Indian culture and traditions. When he reviewed this book and offered valuable suggestions, many a time, it changed the course of my writing for the better.

I thank the rural women of India, whose steadfast faith in the cultural practices around menstruation resulted in these practices being preserved through the sands of time. Ten years ago, I set out to villages as a menstrual educator, thinking that I will teach them; instead, I ended up learning from them.

To the adolescent girls who were never satisfied with my dismissal of menstrual practices as superstition, I remain in debt. If not for their persistent questions, I may never have taken this journey.

I remain grateful to the thousands of readers of my blog, www.mythrispeaks.wordpress.com, through whom I realized the importance of this subject with every write-up that they read and shared. Their questions, experiences, and answers continue to help me deepen my understanding of this subject.

To Bhaskar, who never lost his patience in spite of my persistent questioning of our culture and traditions, and who accompanied me in all my journeys to deepen my understanding; to dear Vyjayanti ji, who always supported and accompanied me even when she couldn't fully understand what I was up to; to Vikshut, Neethu, and Sravanthi, who came on board, no-questions-asked—to all of you, my dear team—I remain grateful for your unconditional support and faith in this work. Often, people long to have at least one person who understands and supports their work. I am immensely grateful that I have had so many.

And to the Grace that made it possible for me, little me, to grasp and share this deep wisdom, I can only bow in servitude.

PART I

MENSTRUATION IN SCIENCE

समग्रं दुःखमायत्तमविज्ञाने द्वयाश्रयम् ।
सुखं समग्रं विज्ञाने विमले च प्रतिष्ठितम् ॥

- च. सू. ३०, ८४

"All ills of humanity are rooted in ignorance
and all progress and happiness in unclouded knowledge."

– Caraka Saṃhitā

Introduction to Part I:

What is Ancient Science?

Evidence

If there is one word that sums up our connection to modern science and all matters scientific, it is evidence. Modern science prides itself on only accepting things that can be proven with evidence. The lack of evidence has come to mean that there is no truth in what is being said. The more the human race moves away from understanding itself, the more it must rely on external evidence to validate its experiences.

For the first five years of my work as a menstrual educator, every time I heard about menstrual practices among rural women, I dismissed them as superstition because of the lack of external evidence. After all, where are the studies which show that menstruating women will be negatively affected if they do not practice seclusion or visit a temple or cook food or touch the tulasī plant while on their period?

But there was always a nagging question which I would not allow to float to the top of my conscious thinking for a long time—how could it be that for thousands of years, millions of women across India have held on to these practices if it is only superstition? That small slit of doubt eventually snowballed into something bigger, enabling me to begin listening to the women. I mean, really listening to them and not just projecting my own thoughts and opinions on to their answers.

Experience

Eventually, I allowed myself to acknowledge my own lack of comprehension and experience of cultural practices around menstruation. And that is when it occurred to me—what the women are sharing as menstrual practices are not just traditions passed down the generations but direct experiences. So, when they say 'we must not go to the temple during menstruation', one among them has seen, heard, or experienced how visiting the temple while menstruating can cause menstrual difficulties. For sure, there have been rebels among women who have broken the rulebook and experienced the outcomes. In close-knit rural communities, such experiences travel like the wind, warning everyone in its path of the ills that come from breaking tradition. As time passes, the stories blur but the warnings remain.

While my newfound methods of unbiased and open listening opened up a world of menstrual practices that I was previously oblivious of, it was my own first-hand experience that made me sit back and take these practices seriously. I realized that the education system I had accepted had conditioned and deeply ingrained in me the need to look only for external evidence. What it did not teach me was that evidence could also come from within, from direct experience.

This is not to say that one must not pursue external research on menstrual practices; by all means, go ahead. But to re-search something, we first need to know what it is that we are searching for. The absence of relevant studies on menstrual practices is because we do not realize that these practices have a purpose. If we did, we would know what to search for. And the truest method of knowing something is by experiencing it first-hand.

However, the problem with experiencing something is that if we do not have the language to express it, it might as well have not happened. For example, during my childhood and teenage years, I constantly suffered from excess body heat. It got worse during summer, when my skin would flare up and my body would feel feverish. But every time I brought this up with an allopathic doctor, they would dismiss it, saying that I have no temperature and so no reason to feel heat. It is only when I was introduced to Āyurved in my thirties that I finally began to understand what I had been going through.

Unlike modern medicine, which only recognizes the measurable quality of temperature, Āyurved has a good understanding of internal heat, which it calls pitta, referring to the internal fire that is crucial for all transformative processes such as metabolism and digestion. In my case, when my Āyurved practitioner did my nāḍīparīkṣā[1], I was told that my prakṛti (body constitution) was largely comprised of pitta. My internal fire was so aggravated that it was burning me up. The associated problems of anger, short temper, sensitive skin, premature graying, and excessive thirst suddenly made sense. The lifestyle changes, yōg, and prāṇāyāma practices I follow post this revelation give me much relief. I feel equally relieved simply knowing that my experience was not imagined and that it had a name and a language in which it could be explained.

Unlike modern science, which does not consider individual experience as 'scientific' evidence, in indigenous science, this gaining of knowledge through direct perception and experience is a method recognized and referred to as pratyakṣa pramāṇa. It is considered as a valid proof of knowledge and reasoning.

Understanding ancient science

To be able to explain menstrual practices that have existed for thousands of years, we need the language of the ancient indigenous sciences and therein starts the difficulty. Indian knowledge systems like Āyurved, Cakra, or even Yōg are not included in India's primary or secondary education curriculum. And worse still, these native sciences are considered as an 'alternative system' which needs to piggyback on modern science to be accepted. I am not saying this out of a possessive feeling toward native science. I am saying this because there is a practical difficulty in comprehending and explaining indigenous medical science like Āyurved through the lens of modern medical science.

The more we learn about varied approaches to science, the more we will realize that science is one. The difference lies in the depth of understanding. Indian knowledge systems understand the human system at the level of the sūkṣma śarīra (subtle body), while modern science works at the level of sthūla śarīra (gross physical body). Consequently, while systems such as Āyurved can often understand and accommodate modern science, the reverse is quite difficult, if not impossible. To understand why, let us take a closer look at the Indian medical system of Āyurved, its origin, and how it is different from modern medical systems.

Origin of Āyurved

A European menstrual researcher once told me that Āyurved is too religious to be considered as a science, and hence she felt hesitant to consider it as a valid means of explaining culturally centered menstrual practices, as I had suggested. I suppose many others too feel that Āyurved is the book of Hindus and is deeply ingrained in Hindu religious thought. It is only natural that such a conclusion will be arrived at by those who are unfamiliar with the Hindu philosophy and sciences like Āyurved, despite such systems being universal in thought and application.

That Hinduism is a way of life, which encompasses a deeper understanding of nature and living systems, is in itself hardly understood by non-Hindus. By attributing its philosophies and sciences to just religious faith, we lose out on the opportunity to tap into a living, breathing system that is perhaps among the very few ancient systems that can still teach us to go back to mother nature and tap into the intelligence inherent in living systems.

From my experience of working with people from different religions across India, I have observed that the Hindu philosophy of life and way of living are very much alive in the culture of the land we call India, even among those who belong to other religious denominations. Therefore, when I use the term 'Hindu' in this book (especially in Part I), unless otherwise mentioned, I am referring to the people who follow this ancient way of living and philosophy, and not just the religion that Hinduism has come to be associated with.

To fully appreciate the logical and scientific methodology applied in Āyurved and get familiarized with the ancient Indian thought process, it is useful to have a basic understanding of the Hindu systems of philosophy, which form the foundation of many ancient Indian texts, including Āyurved. There are six systems of Hindu philosophy called the Ṣaḍ-Darśana. Darśana is derived from 'drś', meaning 'to view'. Ṣaḍ/Ṣat refers to the number six. Darśana refers to the ancient Hindu treatises which provide insights into the physics and metaphysics of creation.

The Ṣaḍ-Darśana aimed at explaining the theory of causation, the purpose of human existence, and also developed the logical reasoning process through which one can arrive at answers to existential questions, find methods to rule out the untruth, and thereby arrive at the truth. Each of these systems was developed by Indian seers (ṛṣi) who spent their entire lives contemplating the nature of truth, with no hidden motive except to alleviate the suffering of mankind and lead them to the path of spiritual liberation.

The Ṣaḍ-Darśana or the six systems of Hindu philosophy are named as Sāṃkhya, Yōg, Nyāya, Vaiśeṣika, Mīmāmsā, and Vedānta. Of these, Mīmāmsā and Vedānta pertain to the religious practices and spiritual thought processes as contained in the Vedas; they can be considered to be outside the scope of this work. The other four systems have contributed to Āyurved in important ways and influenced the scientific and logical approach to the Indian system of medicine. A summary of how the darśanas might have influenced the development of Āyurved is given below.

Sāṃkhya darśana lays down three pramāṇas (proof of knowledge) as reliable methods to arrive at the correct knowledge. These methods are pratyakṣa (perception), anumāna (inference), āptavacana (testimony from a reliable source)[2] and are mentioned in the Āyurved text Caraka saṃhitā as scientific methods for obtaining facts about the patient being treated. In addition, Caraka added yukti, meaning rationale or common sense, as the fourth pramāṇa. [3]

Yōg Sūtras of Patanjali might have played an important role in arriving at the knowledge of the sūkṣma śarīra (anatomy of the subtle body), which forms the basis of understanding the human body as per Āyurved. The Yōg Sūtras mention the process called Saṃyama, which is a mastered technique of combining dhāraṇā (focusing the mind), dhyān (meditation), and samādhi (cessation of activities of the mind).[4] When practiced by a Yōgi, such methods can be used for deepening the understanding of any subject, including the human system. It is probably the reason why the great teachers of Āyurved such as Caraka, Suśruta, and in fact, most scholars of ancient India were ṛṣis (seers).

Nyāya darśana, which is the system of logical reasoning and critical thinking, also has four pramāṇas, which include the three mentioned in Sāṃkhya darśana and a fourth called upamāna (comparison).[5] These four methods of arriving at the correct knowledge based on the physical experience of things are likely to have been made use of in the study of the action of various drugs included in Āyurved.

Vaiśeṣika Sūtras of Kaṇāda propounds two important aspects—one, of describing fundamental substances (padārtha), and two, the atomic model of the universe. Āyurved's classification and understanding of drugs through their inherent rasa (taste) and study of the effect of drugs based on the guṇa (quality) are likely to be based on the knowledge of padārtha. Caraka Saṃhita mentions 57 combinations and

63 types of variations of rasa according to dravya (substance), place, and time.[3]

The most important contribution of Vaiśeṣika philosophy to Āyurved is the atomic theory of creation. Vaiśeṣika philosophy considers the universe as composed of ultimate atoms. According to Vaiśeṣiks, the physical universe is composed of four types of mahābhūtas or bhūta-dravya (fundamental substances or ultimate atoms), which are pṛthvi (earth), agni (fire), āpās (water), and vāyu (air). Ākāśa (ether), which is the fifth mahābhūta, is not included among these. The mahābhūtas are said to exist independent of each other, until creation starts. These fundamental 'ultimate atoms' are said to be indivisible and eternal.

When two of these ultimate atoms (aṇu) combine, they become paramāṇu. When three of these paramāṇu combine, it is called tryaṇuka (triad). It is only then that it becomes perceptible to the senses. Otherwise, aṇu and paramāṇu cannot be perceived. The entire universe has these three types of atoms, i.e. single atoms, twin atoms, and six atoms.[6] Herein lie the fundamentals of Āyurved's theory of tridoṣa of vāta, pitta, and kapha, which are said to be the combination of the mahābhūtas, with vāta predominantly having the qualities of air, pitta predominantly having the qualities of fire, and kapha having the qualities of earth and water. The entire science of Āyurved rests on the principle of the tridoṣa and the knowledge of the indivisible ultimate atoms. (Note that the English translations of these works refer to the mahābhūtas as 'ultimate atoms which are indivisible', indicating that it is not Newtonian atoms, but rather subatomic particles/waves as discovered later in quantum physics). A more detailed explanation of the four darśanas is provided in the section on Notes titled 'Darśana', for the interested reader.

Thus, the origin of Āyurved was influenced by the darśanas, based on a process of scientific inquiry and logical reasoning that were built on the subatomic understanding of creation, considering the human system at the level of the sūkṣma śarīra. It is this deep understanding of the human system at the subtle level that makes Āyurved extremely competent in understanding the root cause of disease and providing methods of preventing disease by weaving this knowledge into cultural practices that became a part and parcel of day-to-day life. Therefore, Āyurved is not just a system of medicine, but the science of life and a way of living.

Fundamental difference between modern medicine and Āyurved

The current understanding of the human system in modern medicine is a biochemical model based on Newtonian classical physics (pre-1900), which generally dealt with macroscopic objects and the forces governing them (Jayasundar 2009, 2011). According to classical physics, the universe can be broken down into atoms, and consequently, the human body too came to be viewed as being composed of atoms as the basic building blocks. Atoms combine together to form molecules, which in turn group to form cells; the cells in turn form tissues. Tissues group to form organs, which in turn create the various systems such as circulatory system, respiratory system, excretory system, etc.

This view created a compartmentalized understanding of the human body, and consequently, several specialties emerged, each functioning independent of the rest. The strict lines drawn between mental health and physical health as independent specializations as a result of such a view has led to undermining the role of the mind in health and well-being. Modern medicine understands the human body as a sum of parts and believes that by studying each part, the whole body can be understood.

Further, disease in modern medicine is understood at the molecular level, and treatment is aimed at the symptoms, with drugs that work to substitute natural bio-chemicals with synthetic ones. Due to this molecular view of disease, the causes of most diseases have not been understood fully. We see this especially when it comes to menstruation—be it dysmenorrhea (period pain), menorrhagia (heavy menstrual bleeding), or more complex conditions like endometriosis, the root cause of these problems is neither understood nor treated. In this system, prevention is more or less ruled out because the cause itself is largely unknown.

Unlike biology, classical physics underwent a major shift when quantum mechanics took over in the early 1900s. The surety of Newtonian atomic and molecular theory fell apart as quantum physics ventured into the area of subatomic particles and declared that at the subatomic level, particles can exist simultaneously as particles and waves. Heisenberg, the architect of quantum mechanics, said, "Underlying all physical matter is the intrinsically interconnected dynamic network of energy leaving nothing isolated in the universe." Essentially, it means that all of us and everything around us is made up of waves of energy, and we are all interconnected and influence each other. This is called the quantum worldview, which replaced the earlier worldview proposed by Newton. However, modern medicine is yet to boldly venture into quantum biology for diagnosis and treatment of diseases, and it continues to be satisfied with the old method of symptom suppression and treatment of parts in isolation.

Āyurved is based on the subatomic understanding of the human body. In other words, quantum biology. Consequently, there is no compartmentalization of biological systems or separation of mental and physical health. Here, the whole is inclusive of the parts, and the parts are understood to be in continuous interaction with the whole. In Āyurved, disease is understood at the subtle level of what causes the molecular disturbance and chemical imbalance in the human body, through the influence of the subtle forces called tridoṣa, which control various functions within the body. A comprehensive understanding of the tridoṣa system will help to understand the root cause of disease. Treatment is, therefore, not targeted at the molecular level, but at the subatomic level where the cause first arose, while taking into consideration the role played by the mind as well as the environment.

Although Āyurved was based on the knowledge of the sūkṣma śarīra, it did not shy away from practicing and teaching surgery. The surgical techniques that were discovered by Suśruta are said to have laid the foundation for modern surgery in Europe. Suśruta discovered the art of cataract-crouching, which was unknown to the surgeons of ancient Greece and Egypt. Limbs were amputated; abdominal sections were performed; fractures were set; dislocations, hernia, and ruptures were reduced; hemorrhoids and fistula were removed. Suśruta's work on practical midwifery was really ahead of its time and is probably the first text which mentions Cesarean sections in cases where natural delivery is ruled out or if the fetus has died in the womb[7]. The transplanting of sensible skin-flaps is also entirely an Indian method. It is Suśruta who first successfully demonstrated the feasibility of mending a clipped earlobe with a patch of sensible skin-flap scraped from the neck or the adjoining part. Ackernecht has aptly observed in his book A Short History of Medicine:

"There is little doubt that plastic surgery in Europe which flourished in medieval Italy is a direct descendant of classical Indian surgery."[8]

While Āyurved, with its understanding of how the human body functions at the level of the sūkṣma śarīra as well as the sthūla śarīra, can very well understand and accommodate modern medicine, the reverse is not possible until and unless modern medicine deepens its understanding of the human body beyond atoms and molecules and enters the realm of the sūkṣma śarīra. Though ancient, India's native sciences are far more advanced through their subtlety, compared to the modern scientific understanding of biology and medicine. A quantum theory-based treatment is the next level of evolution for modern medicine, which is waiting to happen. And once it does, doctors will be able to prevent and treat menstrual disorders (and other diseases) with far greater success, just as Āyurved currently does.

Similarity between Āyurved and other ancient medical systems

The earliest texts of Āyurved are said to have been compiled somewhere around 6th century B.C.[9] But the knowledge contained in Āyurved is likely to have existed years before it was formally codified. Even according to modern historians, the mention of various methods of healing is found in the Atharva Veda texts dated around 1200 BC - 1000 BC[10,11]. The earliest written texts of Āyurved are credited to Caraka and are called Caraka Saṃhitā, which is known for its diagnostic excellence and therapeutics. A later text by Suśruta called Suśruta Saṃhitā is known for its knowledge of anatomy and is the earliest recorded information on surgical procedures, including plastic surgery.

When we study ancient sciences from different parts of the world, we can hardly ignore the many similarities of philosophies and science that emerged in ancient India and in the early Western, Arab, and Asian civilizations, before the emergence of Western medicine or allopathy as we know it today. A glimpse into the similarities between Āyurved and other ancient sciences in different regions of the world is presented below.

Hippocrates & humoral pathology

The period of Āyurved precedes that of Hippocrates (circa 460–377 BC) by about 150 years. The similarity between Āyurved's tridoṣa system and Hippocrates' humoral pathology is often discussed. Some accounts mention that Hippocrates was influenced by the tridoṣa system, perhaps through the knowledge of Āyurved brought to Greece by Pythagoras, who is said to have traveled to India and learned from Buddhist masters. [12] The borrowing of Āyurved's knowledge by the Greek is also mentioned by Dr. Wise[13] in Review of the History of Medicine:

> "Hippocrates, the "father of medicine", borrowed his materia medica from the Hindus. When the Greeks visited

India in the fourth century, they found the Hindus proficient in the art of healing, and Alexander the Great kept Hindu physicians in his camp for the treatment of diseases which Greek physicians could not heal." [14]

In comparing Hippocrates' humoral pathology to Āyurved's tridoṣa system, Berdoe says[15]:

"What is known as the Humoral Pathology formed the most essential part of the system of the Dogmatics. Humoral Pathology explains all diseases as caused by the mixture of the four cardinal humours, viz., the blood, bile, mucus or phlegm and water. Hippocrates first leaned towards it, but it was Plato who developed it."

In Āyurved, the tridoṣa are called as vāta, pitta, and kapha. Further, Āyurved recognizes the role of rakta (blood) along with the tridoṣa in the maintenance of bodily functions, though it was not included as the fourth humor. However, Āyurved is clear that pitta is not bile, just as kapha is not phlegm. Hippocrates' humoral pathology seems to have replaced pitta with bile and kapha with phlegm, while leaving out vāta, which is the most important doṣa, as it corresponds to the nervous system and influences the other doṣas as well. Therefore, the humoral pathology of Hippocrates is not the same as Āyurved's tridoṣa system, but there is a similarity in the thought process, which was to understand the human system at a subtle level.

Persian, Arabic & Latin medicine

The works of Caraka and Suśruta were translated into Arabic, under the patronage of Kaliph Almansur, in the 7th century[16]. The translations were said to be made from Saṃskṛtam to Persian and then from Persian to Arabic. Abdullah bin Ali is said to have translated the Caraka Saṃhitā, and Manka was said to be the translator of Suśruta Saṃhitā into Persian.[17] Caraka Saṃhitā was translated into Arabic in the beginning of the 8th century, and it was titled Sharaka Indianus.[18] The Arabic version of Suśruta is known by the name of Kitab-Shaw Shoon-a-Hindi or Kitab-i-Susrud. Similarly, Aṣṭāṅgahṛdaya of Vagbhata was translated as Kitāb Ashtānkar. A reference to this has been made in Firdaus al-Hikmah.[16] Ibn Abi Usaybia devotes an entire chapter to physicians from India in his book Uyun al-Anba fi Tabaqat al-Atibba, where he mentions the names of two Indian translators Manka and Ibn Dhann, 12 Indian works of medicine that were translated into Arabic, 19 Indian physicians, and 25 titles of books.[17]

The name of Caraka occurs in the Latin translation of Avicenna (Ibn Sina), the Iranian philosopher and physician of the 10th and 11th centuries. His concept of humoral theory is closer to Āyurved than it is to the Hippocratic concept. Several of the drugs he prescribed such as Itrephal is nothing but Triphala of Ayurvedic texts. On several occasions, he mentioned Hubbul Hind, meaning 'Indian Pill', Jawarishul Hind, meaning 'Indian curnam', and Majanul Hind, meaning 'Indian leham', to give a few examples.[19] Similarly, we find mention of evidence of the influence of Indian medicine in the works of other famous physicians like Rhazes (Al Razi) and Serapion (Ibn Serabi).

The first European translation of Suśruta Saṃhitā was published by Dr. Franciscus Hessler in Latin as Susrutas Ayurvedas in 1844 and by Muller in German in the early 19th century. The Latin versions are said to have formed the basis of European medicine. [20]

Similarities between homeopathy and Āyurved

Of the newer systems of medicine that emerged in Europe, homeopathy (introduced in the late 1700s) bears a striking resemblance to Āyurved in its fundamental understanding of disease and well-being. Founded by the German Physician Dr. Sameul Hanhemann, disease in homeopathy is understood and treated at the subtle level of the 'vital force'. According to Dr. Hanhemann, "Every disease (not entirely surgical) consists only in a special, morbid, dynamic alteration of our vital energy." The term vital force is well understood in India as prāṇa. The acceptance and continued practice of homeopathy in India is possibly due to our ease of understanding the concept of prāṇa and treatment aimed at the prāṇic body.

Similarities between Āyurved and Traditional Chinese Medicine (TCM)

The movement of Buddhist monks from India to China in the 1st century AD is well documented and known to have led to the initiation of cultural exchange between these two nations, with the knowledge of medicine playing a prominent role in these exchanges. Buddhist monks, who were trained in medicine as part of their initiation, are known to have extended their medical knowledge to the Chinese. Records indicate that many Chinese Buddhist monks studied in the ancient Indian universities such as Nalanda. Chinese medical works and pharmacopeia from the 5th century AD onwards include materials suggesting connections with Buddhist medicine that resemble Āyurved. Two works on ophthalmology attributed to Nāgārjuna[21] exist in Chinese medicine, and they were important standard works studied by the students of ophthalmology in China till the 16th century AD. Similarly, there exists much information about the introduction of ophthalmic knowledge from China into Japan through the Buddhists.[22]

Writings of Tao Hongjing (456-536 AD), a famous medical writer, alchemist, and pharmacologist, depicted the influence of Buddhists' four elements theory Si da for the first time. One of the articles in Chinese Buddhist canon translates the tridoṣa as follows: vāta – 'feng', meaning wind, pitta – 'huang', meaning yellow, kapha – 'tan', meaning phlegm.[22] These might be the reasons for the many similarities between Traditional Chinese Medicine (TCM) and Āyurved, as given in the below examples.

Āyurved's marma points and the Chinese acupuncture pressure points are remarkably similar. TCM considers four bodily humors – qi, blood, moisture, and essence. The Chinese knowledge of qi finds much resemblance to the Indian understanding of prāṇa, while blood has the properties of pitta, moisture of kapha, and essence of vāta. The concepts of yin and yang as the opposite yet complimentary and interdependent energies are similar to the Indian concepts of prakṛti and puruṣa. TCM considers water, earth, metal, wood, and fire as the five elements of the material world, while Indian science considers earth, fire, water, air, and ether as the five elements or pañca mahābhūta.

Apart from the ancient sciences mentioned above, there are many other examples such as that of the medicine men and women of Native America called Shamans, whose concepts and practices have a resemblance to that of the ancient Hindus. Similarly, the healing science of Japan called reiki is about channelizing the prāṇa, known as ki among Japanese, to treat patients.

Although these are just a few examples that could be covered within the limited scope of this book, it is enough to give us an idea of the intermixing of ancient sciences and how there must have been a similar understanding of fundamental principles and subtle sciences across the world. Decoding the cultural practices of a region without an understanding of their ancient science would, therefore, be an incomplete and, perhaps, futile attempt.

Decline of Indian and other ancient sciences

During the Mahomedan rule (A.C. 1001 – 1707), Indian medicine began to decline, due to lack of governmental support, as well as the turmoil and unrest spread across the country owing to the invasions. During this period, the world's earliest universities which were established in India, such as Tākṣaśila and Nālanda, were destroyed. It is said that nine million books were burned in Nālanda for three months by Bakhtiyar Khilji in 1193. The Indian medical sciences showed signs of revival briefly during the time of the Peshwas (A.C. 1715 - 1818), and some of the most recent works on Indian medicine were compiled during this time. However, the Peshwas were overthrown by the British in 1818, and from the fall of the Marathas began the decline of the native medical sciences. The colonizers not only established medical schools and colleges based on their knowledge of medicine (allopathy) but also suppressed the growth and promotion of Indian sciences, depriving the world of ancient knowledge systems.

While Indian sciences suffered destruction at the hands of invaders and colonizers, the native sciences in America and Europe, too, suffered a decline with the spread of Christianity.

The pre-Columbian Native American cultures were significantly impacted from the time of the European invasion, starting in 1492, which introduced Christianity to America. Similarly, who can forget the age of European witch hunts, which lasted for 150 years (starting in the 1550s), where no fewer than 80,000 people were tried for witchcraft and half of them executed.[23] Those who were called witches were very likely the native healers and medicine women of that time.

The origin of modern science

Often, people assume that India's native sciences are applicable only to Hindus, and hence can be ignored by the rest. But the truth remains that there was a time when across the world, similar knowledge systems existed, before it was destroyed through organized crime against those who were traditional scientists and healers; sometimes by burning them at the stake, calling them witches, sometimes dismissing such knowledge as religious belief, and mostly by self-proclaimed elite groups' suppression of such knowledge by terming it pseudo-science. The origin of modern science as we know it is a story that rests on the planned destruction of ancient science and traditional scientists.

In his essay, Jayant ji explains how a few groups of elite men decided what constituted modern science. It started with the setting up of the Royal Society of London for Improving Natural Knowledge by King Charles II in 1661, with Robert Boyle as the founder. Below are a few passages from his essay "An Outsider Deconstructing European Enlightenment: Death in Three Acts".[24]

> "Robert Boyle (1627 - 1691) was looking at ways in which nature could be tamed and dominated through experimentation, and to be able to do so, without engaging different groups of people with multiple, different views on how nature works based on their experiences, that is, by effectively dismissing the traditional knowledge systems."

Traditional folk healers held nature and its connection to humans as sacred, thereby weaving into their culture many aspects that prevented the destruction of nature. But this understanding had to be dismantled if nature had to be exploited for development. And what better way to make this happen than by calling all ancient knowledge systems as unscientific and inaccessible to the medicine men and women of the time. Jayant ji further writes:

> "Robert Boyle was a wealthy feudal aristocrat, the son of the Earl of Cork. Boyle conducted his experiments in his mansion in London to which he invited selected witnesses and reviewers who were of his social class. Thus, began the 'peer reviewed' scientific methodology attested by a few elite, which is what we follow to this day. It provided an inherent advantage to the elite who could afford the laboratory and amongst themselves choose their peers."

To this day, access to scientific methodology, labs, and procedures to publish data, however valid, are cumbersome and available only to a few who are already part of such networks. Worse still is the mandate that requires all sciences to fit within the limited framework of modern science in order to be considered valid. What we have at the end of the day is summarized well by Jayant ji below:

> "The result of this top down expensive laboratory-based science was production and deployment of complex technology requiring large amounts of capital, targeted at dominating and exploiting nature."

So, when I say 'ancient science', it must be remembered that what is presented in this book is not something exclusive to a certain set of people in a specific land but is the very essence of the traditional knowledge systems which understood life in its subtility and worked in tandem with nature but was lost to humanity at some point in history.

In India, although much of our native sciences and knowledge were systematically destroyed by the invaders and colonizers, some of them still remained in documented form, and many were later revived and re-written by scholars and experts. What is presented in this book are insights derived from such texts within the context of India.

It is a bit of a wonder how the women in India, especially the rural grandmothers, have kept alive these ancient knowledge systems through their cultural practices in the most unsuspecting subject of menstruation. It was the place where nobody thought to look, and therefore, it survived to this date.

References for Introduction to Part 1

1. Nāḍīparīkṣā refers to Āyurved's diagnosis method through pulse reading
2. Sinha, Nandalal. The Sacred Book of the Hindus, Vol X1, Samkhya Philosophy, 1915
3. Sharma P.V., Caraka Samhita, Volume 1, Revised edition, 2014
4. Prasada, Rama. The Sacred Book of the Hindus, Vol IV, The Yōga Sūtra of Patanjali, 1924
5. Vidyabhusana, Satish Chandra. The Sacred Book of the Hindus, Vol VIII, The Nyāya Sūtra of Gotama, 1930
6. Sinha, Nandalal. The Sacred Book of the Hindus, Vol VI, The Vaiśeṣika Sūtra of Kaṇāda, 1923
7. Kaviraj Kunja Lal Bhishagratna, An English Translation of Sushruta Samhita, Vol 1 – Suthrasthanam, 1907
8. Ackernecht EH. A short history of medicine. Johns Hopkins University Press.1955
9. Saini, A. Physicians of Ancient India, 2016
10. Michael Witzel (2003), "Vedas and Upaniṣads", in The Blackwell Companion to Hinduism (Editor: Gavin Flood), Blackwell, page 68
11. M. S. Valiathan. The Legacy of Caraka. Orient Blackswan. page. 22.
12. E. Pococke, India in Greece, 2014
13. Dr. Wise, Review of the History of Medicine, 1867

14. H. H. Sir Bhagvat Sinh JEE (Thakur Saheb of Gondal) A Short History of Aryan Medical Science, 1896
15. Berdoe, Edward. The Origin and Growth of The Healing Art, 1893
16. Chari P.S. Sushruta and our heritage. Indian Journal of plastic surgery, 2003
17. Khan M.S. An Arabic Source for the History of Ancient Indian Medicine. Indian Journal of History of Science 16 (1): 47 - 56, May 1981
18. Hunter, W.W. The Indian Empire: Its People. History and Products, 1886
19. Bag, A.K. Ibn Sina and Indian Science. Indian Journal of History of Science, 21(3): 270 - 275 (1986)
20. Thamburaj, Vincent A. Textbook of Contemporary Neurosurgery, 2012
21. Nāgārjuna is an important contributor to ancient Āyurved and is known as the person who revised Suśruta Saṃhita
22. Deshpande, Vijaya Jayant. Glimpses of Ayurveda in Medieval Chinese Medicine. Indian Journal of History of Science, 43.2 (2008) 137-161
23. Leeson, Peter T and Russ, Jacob W. The Witch-Trials
24. Kalawar, Jayant. An Outsider Deconstructing European Enlightenment: Death in Three Acts. 2019
25. Waghmare Sachin S, Mhaiskar Bhushan D, Darshanik Background Of Ayurveda, International Ayurvedic Medical Journal. Volume 2;Issue 3; May - June 2014. ISSN: 23205091

26. Jayasundar R. Quantum physics, Ayurveda and spirituality. In: Mishra SC, editor. Science and Spirituality Quest. Kolkata, India: National Institute of Technology and Bhaktivedanta Institute; 2008. pp. 11–28.

27. Advent of a Link between Ayurveda and Modern Health Science: The Proceedings of the First International Congress on Ayurveda, "Ayurveda: The Meaning of Life—Awareness, Environment, and Health" March 21-22, 2009, Milan, Italy Antonio Morandi, Carmen Tosto, [...], and Paolo Roberti di Sarsina

28. Sanjeev Rastogi. Building bridges between Ayurveda and Modern Science, International Journal of Ayurveda Research, 2010 Jan-Mar; 1(1): 41–46.

कृत्स्नो हि लोको बुद्धिमतामाचार्यः शत्रुश्चाबुद्धिमताम्

"The entire world is the teacher to the intelligent and foe to the unintelligent."

– (Caraka Saṃhitā)

CHAPTER 1

MENARCHE: THE NEED FOR CELEBRATION

During one of my workshops for urban college-going women, something unexpected happened. A young woman who was listening to me suddenly became unconscious and slumped on her chair. What followed was a flurry of activities trying to help her, and someone arranged to take her to a medical examination room in the college. When she became conscious, I asked her what had happened to cause such a reaction in her. Her friends suggested that it might be because she hadn't eaten. But she shook her head in negation, looked right at me and said, "It's blood. When someone repeatedly talks about blood, I can't handle it. I pass out."

While this was a rare and extreme reaction to conversations on menstruation, it is not so rare to come across urban women who feel stressed out every time they menstruate or even hear someone else talk about it. Indeed, this is the reason why many associate menstruation with stigma and generalize that all women in India associate menstruation with a negative attitude. This, of course, is far from the fact.

From my observations on interacting with women across different sections of society and various communities across India, I have found that the attitude toward menstruation has turned negative or indifferent as women moved away from culturally centered ideas of menstruation. Often, I have observed that the rural and tribal women who have not been through a formal education system or have had minimal exposure to the urban way of living exhibit a positive and sometimes (seemingly) exaggerated enthusiasm toward menstruation as nature's or God's gift to women. I recall my conversation with a woman who had never been schooled, asking me to suggest to her some treatment by which she can start menstruating again (she had reached menopause at the time of my interview). To her understanding, menstruation and well-being are synonymous. For many rural women like her, menstruation has to do with good health, and they rarely limit it to childbirth, as we are taught in the current education system.

Our observations on the variations in attitude toward menstruation were corroborated when my team and I undertook a study (unpublished) of 1035 women across four districts in Karnataka, which included urban women and adolescent girls from Bengaluru and rural women and adolescent girls from villages in districts of Chamarajanagar, Raichur, and Uttara Kannada. We found that overall, 57.77% of those interviewed felt positive about menstruation, 23.38% felt indifferent, and 18.84% had a negative attitude toward menstruation. The majority of women interviewed expressed a positive outlook toward menstruation, breaking the stereotypical assumption that Indian women associate shame with menstruation.

What is noteworthy is that women and girls from urban Bengaluru had the highest percentage of negative attitude (26.69%), as compared to women and girls from rural areas (15.26% to 17.87%). I recall my own interviews with rural women who would smile, sometimes feel shy, but mostly say that menstruation was a positive occurrence in their life. In stark contrast, the urban women I interviewed would arrogantly shoot back a question, asking, "Why on earth would anyone feel positive toward menstruation?"

We need to introspect as to what it is about indigenous knowledge and culture that enabled a positive and reverential attitude toward menstruation, which is so different from the stressful, stigmatized notion that has percolated our mind with modern education and urban lifestyle. The answers start with understanding the approach to menarche, the first period.

Menstrual memory

The memory of the first period can trigger a similar response in subsequent periods. This is thanks to a small part of the brain called the hippocampus, whose job is to store and retrieve memories through our subconscious mind[1]. When a memory is retrieved, our body subconsciously responds to the memory the same way it did the first time. This is termed as episodic memory. For example, we might have experienced instances where perhaps a fragrance sets off a pleasant memory, and a particular location (say, a road where an accident occurred) sets off a stressful reaction to a negative incident. It is the same with menstrual memory. If the experience of the first period was negative and stressful, it is likely that every subsequent period throws the body into a subconscious stress response.

This is one of the reasons why in Indian culture, all efforts are made to ensure that the first period is a happy one, and no stone is left unturned to make the young girl feel special and cherished throughout the menarche celebration.

For those who have had unpleasant memories of menarche, a conscious effort to replace those memories with pleasant instances lies at the core of reducing the stress around menstruation. It is true that many women may not have had much choice about their circumstances as young girls, but as adults, it is in their hands to bring awareness to this aspect of menstrual memory and consciously work to dust the unpleasant cobwebs of past experiences so that their menstrual experience does not become a painful one. Here is an interesting experience shared by a wise woman during a discussion on how the attitude toward menstruation can shape our experience of it:

"I used to suffer from painful periods until I turned 40 years of age. One particular month, I was down with severe pain and was frustrated. I shared this with a female friend and told her that I am unable to handle this every month. She then shared a few wise words with me, which completely changed the way I experienced my period. She told me to be thankful and grateful for my uterus, which is the creative Śakti (primordial feminine creative force) in me, and to repeat that to myself whenever I feel pain. The day I accepted this wisdom and learned to be grateful to my uterus, my pain vanished. From that day onwards, the moment I wake up each morning, I sit in silence for five minutes and thank my uterus for the blessings received, for making me a mom twice."

Traditional understanding of health

Āyurved stresses on the individual's ability to shape his/her health based on his/her thought process. It is agreed in modern medicine as well that stress negatively impacts the physical well-being, resulting in psychosomatic disorders (diseases of the mind that affect the body). The influence of the mind on creating disease of the body is explained in the Upanishad[2], through the knowledge of pañcakośa or five sheaths that make the human body. These sheaths include the physical body but also extend beyond it, as follows:

- Annamaya kośa – the gross or physical kośa, which sustains on the food consumed
- Prāṇamaya kośa – the vital kośa resulting from breathing and flow of prāṇa (vital life force)
- Manomaya kośa – the mind-based kośa, with thoughts which cause mental modifications
- Vijñānamaya kośa – the intelligence kośa, where the mind has gained the ability to distinguish right from wrong (vijñāna)
- Ānandamaya kośa – the eternal bliss kośa that results in enlightenment

A person who exists in the ānandamaya kośa is the spiritually enlightened one; suffering does not touch such a one. This level of existence is reached by those who practice intense sādhana (spiritual practice) and whose awareness resides in the ānandamaya kośa. An example of this is of the great sage Śrī Ramana Maharshi, who was diagnosed with bone cancer but never asked for treatment, nor till the last breath did he express pain or suffering.

Those who exist in the vijñānamaya kośa will have the capacity to prevent mental modifications by their ability to discern right from wrong and thus prevent it from affecting the manomaya and other kośas. Meditation techniques play an important role in strengthening this layer and preventing mental disturbances that might manifest physically at a later stage. The many ailments owing to mental stress and emotional turmoil are examples of the inability to rest our awareness in the vijñānamaya kośa.

For most of us, problems begin at the manomaya kośa or, simply put, the mind. With every event that happens, our emotions get the better of us, and consequently, we are consumed by stress. Stressful thoughts, in turn, affect our breathing patterns and thereby impact the prāṇamaya kośa. If we observe how the pace and manner of breathing change during stress, happiness, and instances of deep relaxation, we will understand the play of the prāṇamaya kośa. When stress begins to impact breathing patterns, prāṇayama or breathing techniques can play a very important role to regulate the breath and prevent it from disturbing the annamaya kośa. If the prāṇamaya kośa is affected, it eventually manifests as disease in the annamaya kośa or physical body. At this stage, treatment becomes necessary.

The reverse, that is, the diseases manifesting in the annamaya kośa affecting the other kośa, is also possible. These are called somatopsychic diseases, referring to the disease of the physical body causing problems in mental health. For example, recent studies have shown that gut bacteria can have an effect on mental health.[3]

While the celebratory nature of menarche rituals ensures a positive outlook toward menstruation, the other traditional practices followed during menarche have a direct impact on the physical and mental health of the menstruating girl. The interconnections between physical and mental health, especially with respect to menstruation, are well understood in Āyurved. It will not be an exaggeration to state that a woman's menstrual health is only as good as her mental health and vice versa.

Girls and women who have followed menarche rituals swear by its efficacy in preventing menstrual disorders even later in life. Due to this understanding, often, mothers go out of their way to organize the menarche celebration for their daughters, even if it means taking a financial loan.

History of menarche celebration in India

The cultural celebration of menarche among Hindus still continues in much of South India and in some North-Eastern states like Assam and Manipur. In Central and Northern India, unfortunately, such practices no longer exist, partly because of the Muslim invasion and partly because menarche celebration was tied to the early marriage of the girl child.

With the invasion of the Muslim rulers in North India, the celebration of menarche came to a halt, as families became wary of announcing the eligibility of young girls to the rulers, who would often misbehave with them or take them away. When child marriage was in existence, even after marriage, the young bride would continue to stay in her parents' house until she attained menarche. Then, with a ritualistic celebration called gauṇa, she would be taken to her husband's home. Many

North Indian families continue to celebrate gauṇa as part of the marriage ceremony even now, wondering why the adult bride has to ritualistically go to her parents' house and then return! Later, with the abolishment of child marriage, the practice of gauṇa as a menarche ritual ended altogether. The absence of menarche celebration in Northern India is one of the reasons why women might have lost the positive association with menstruation in these regions.

Where it does exist, menarche celebrations are nothing short of a marriage function, and they begin soon after the first period. What is most interesting is how the Hindu culture encompassed all that we try to package today as 'Menstrual Education' in a much more loving and comprehensive manner, with practical lessons on how to manage one's period and a diet that would aid the adolescent girl's well-being during this crucial time. The knowledge transferred during this process went way beyond superficial menstrual hygiene associated with particular products and included practices that prevent menstrual disorders, traditional ways of honoring the feminine within, and teaching young girls to respect their body as they entered womanhood.

Overview of menarche rituals

Menarche celebration is one of the rites of passage for young Hindu girls who attain puberty. It is generally termed ṛtu kāla saṃskāra, with celebrations varying from 11 to 16 days. Based on the cultural diversities, different names and variations in practices have emerged. Most of these practices are handed down orally through generations of grandmothers and are difficult to trace back to codified texts. It is likely that these practices were customized for each region based on the availability of food, type of environment, and knowledge of medicine in each community, resulting in the many diverse practices. It is incredible that this knowledge system survived solely through the efforts of generations of Indian women, with no formal documentation.

A few of the practices in different states based on first-hand information I gathered during conversations with the practitioners are presented below. The scientific explanations of the practices as per my understanding are provided in the next sub-heading.

In Karnataka, the celebration is colloquially called hosige or ārati (waving of lighted lamps). The practice is also called soppu hākodu, which directly refers to the menstrual hut built for the menstruating girl. In the districts of Dharward and Bijapur, one of the special nutritious preparations for the menarche celebration is antina unde, a sweet laddu made with dry fruits such as dates, raisins, almonds, cashew nut, along with ghee (clarified butter) and the gum/resin of babul (Acacia) tree. From the first day of the period, a menstrual hut is built in the backyard, and the menstruating girl is welcomed to stay and rest in the hut. The hut is made of coconut leaves, mango leaves, and specific medicinal plants, such as neem, which help to prevent aggravation of the doṣas and protect the menstruating girl through their anti-bacterial, anti-inflammatory, and other medicinal properties, since her immunity is considered to be low during menstruation.

Among the Pillai and Mudaliar communities in Tamil Nadu, where it is called poopu naniraattu vizha, the raw egg yolk of a country chicken is poured in half a glass of sesame oil or ghee and the girl is asked to swallow it whole. The egg is said to contain the same nutrients that her body produces and therefore believed to aid the process of menstruation. Ghee offsets the pitta (heat-inducing) properties of egg and soothes the digestive system. Urad dal (black gram) and sesame are also considered as good sources of calcium, required to strengthen the bones. Here too, a menstrual hut is constructed with coconut/palm leaves for the girl to rest (it might be discontinued among urban families). The rituals are meant to pamper the girl and make her feel special and support her health during this crucial phase of transition.

In the state of Assam, the girl is fed on raw fruits which are easy to digest and help ease menstrual pain and discomfort. This is similar to the haviṣya-anna mentioned in ancient Āyurved texts like Suśruta Saṃhitā. Haviṣya-anna involves eating only fruits, vegetables, and dairy products from cow's milk and is generally prescribed for those who take up intense sādhana (spiritual practice). It is interesting how the diet recommended for sādhana is similar to what is prescribed for menstruating girls.

In Andhra Pradesh, the celebration is called samurta function. The word samurta or samarta means that the girl has become able or able-bodied. Below is a detailed account of the menarche rituals of a Brahmin girl in Andhra Pradesh, as shared by the girl's mother, Smt. Hema Latha Guda. This account is of a menstrual celebration that happened in the year 2016.

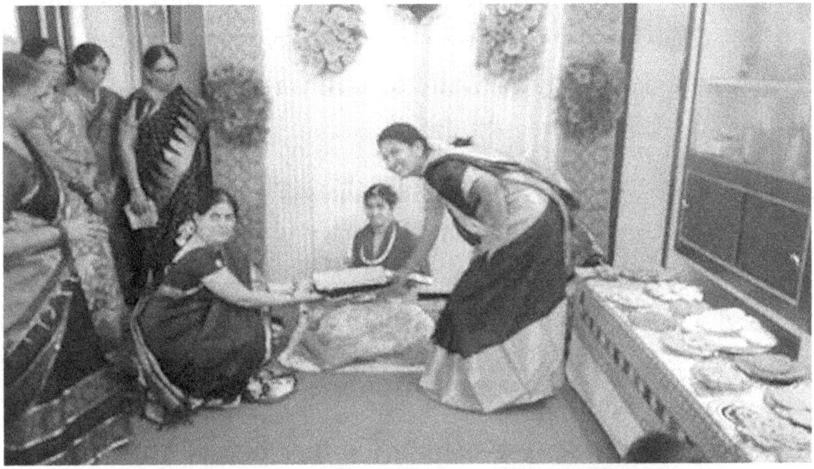

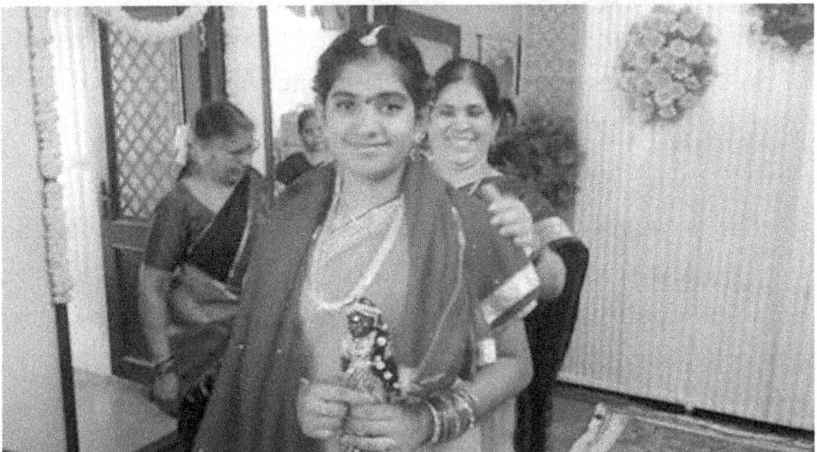

Figure 1 & 2 Menarche ritual of a young girl in Andhra Pradesh, with her mother, grandmother, and aunts

The girl, around the age of 12, upon attaining puberty, is honored to have become a 'grown-up'. After her first menstrual period, she is felicitated by women in the family and the neighborhood, in the form of festivities. If the ruling star of the girl is not auspicious at the time of puberty, then a śānti pūjā is performed according to Vedic rites, after giving a purification bath to the girl on the fifth day.

Soon after the first period starts, a mat is laid in a corner of a room (to ensure privacy). In some places, palm leaves are spread like a mat. On this mat, a clean, white cloth is spread. A red color solution is prepared by mixing turmeric and a pinch of choona (slaked lime/calcium hydroxide) with water. The girl's mother/aunt/grandmother dip their hand in the solution and make hand impressions on the four corners of the white cloth. The girl too makes impressions on the wall with this red water (turmeric + slaked lime). The girl is seated in the middle of the mat, facing east or north. The mat on which the girl sits is called dadiyamu. She is given sweets or dry coconut, jaggery, and sesame for consumption.

She is taught to be clean and tidy. At all times, she has the company of at least one girl or an adult woman. She receives help and counseling regarding the use of cloth/pad, hygiene, and other aspects related to menstruation. The women ensure that she will be kept happy. Many girls cry or weep during this time. If this happens, they are embraced by their mother or grandmother, who tell the girl that it is an auspicious and happy occasion and nothing to worry about.

A word is sent to the girl's maternal grandparents, maternal uncle as well as paternal relatives and family. Neighbors and friends are also informed.

During the menstrual period, the girl is made to rest for 3-5 days, seating her separately so that she does not come into contact with any infectious agency, since her immune system will be weak during menstruation. This practice continues during her subsequent periods as well. The dress that the girl wears on the first day of the first period is given away to the dhobi (washer-man). During the first three days, the girl is not allowed to touch anything. Only her mother/aunt who helps her with the routines touches her, but they take a bath before entering other rooms.

On the evening of the first day, she is given a good bath, and usual śṛṅgāra (make-up) like bindi, kuṅkuma, flowers, bangles, turmeric on the feet, etc. are done. On this day, a perantam is held. Perantam is a practice where married women (suhagan) perform ārati to the girl. Only very close family, friends, and neighbors participate on this day. A tray filled with dry coconut, jaggery, and sesame laddu (a ball of sweet) is given to the girl by one of the suhagans. No expensive gifts are given; only tambulam (betel leaf and araca nut) and mūng dal (green gram) are given to the suhagans. No return gifts are given. Traditional songs are a must and are usually sung by the women. This is a rather private and low-key affair, and it is done for the first four evenings. From the 5th day until the 16th day, the celebrations are more elaborate and extravagant.

Fourth-day bath – At very early hours, turmeric is applied on the girl's body, and she is given a good bath. She comes out of the seclusion room on the 4th day. She is given a drink made with turmeric and water—pasupu theertham—to prevent infection.

Fifth-day bathing ceremony – The girl is given a maṅgal snān, that is, an auspicious bath, on the fifth day. After this, she is entitled to enter the pūjā room also. The women who administer the maṅgal snān to the girl will be gifted a saree.

Dietary recommendations during the first menstrual period include the following:

- No salt and paprika (dry chili powder) for the first three days
- Sesame, dry coconut, and jaggery are a must
- No buttermilk or curd
- Milk is given
- Ghee can be consumed
- Khichidi/Khichiri made with mūng dal (green gram), rice, and ghee should be given. Salt is not added to this preparation. This is given for the first three days
- Plenty of water is given
- Sweets (certain varieties) are also given

Evening celebrations from the 5th to 16th day – Some people end the festivities on the 9th day. On the last day, there will be a grand perantam. The girl is seated on a high chair. She is very well dressed, with lots of bangles, flowers, and ornaments. Sweets are given to the girl, and later, they are displayed. Usually, 11 to 21 varieties of sweets are prepared. Gifts are also given to the girl. Return gifts are given to the suhagans along with tambulum. Each day's expense is sometimes sponsored by one of the close relatives. There will be a very grand celebration on the 16th day, when the expenses are borne only by the parents. The celebrations are done only during the daytime, and festivities are wrapped up in the evening.

In general, the celebrations among the Brahmin community involve only close relatives and few friends, whereas the celebrations in other Hindu communities are more elaborate, resembling the festivities of a marriage.

Decoding the menarche rituals

In spite of the many variations in practices, some aspects are common across regions, and those provide answers to the scientific understanding of these rituals. Most women who follow these practices attribute reasons such as building immunity, increasing calcium and iron intake, strengthening the uterus, and so on. When we look closer at the practices with a scientific lens, we will be surprised at the depth to which menstruation was understood by our ancestors.

Let us begin with the explanations as per modern science. To understand the subtle changes involved during menstruation, we will need to take a closer look at the atomic and cellular changes that occur within the female system during menstruation.

During menstruation, the female body produces more free radicals than usual. Free radicals are known to cause cellular damage, resulting in disease and aging. The excess free radicals throw the body into oxidative stress, which is known to be the reason for primary dysmenorrhea (period pain) and also infertility, unless it is countered by antioxidants. Understanding this phenomenon is crucial to decode many of the menstrual practices during menarche.

Some definitions of terms that will help those who might be unfamiliar with these words are presented in the following paragraphs.

Free radicals

If an atom does not have a full outer shell due to insufficient electrons, it becomes unstable and seeks to bond with another atom, using the electron from the nearby atom to complete its outer shell. The unstable atoms are called free radicals. In the state of being a free radical, the atoms have a positive charge and are also called positive charge ions or cations.

Reactive oxygen species (ROS)

There are many types of radicals, but those of most concern in biological systems are derived from oxygen and are known collectively as reactive oxygen species. Oxygen has two unpaired electrons in separate orbitals in its outer shell. This electronic structure makes oxygen especially susceptible to radical formation.

Oxidative stress

When oxygen molecules split into single atoms that have unpaired electrons, they become unstable free radicals that seek other atoms or molecules to bond to. If this continues to happen, it begins a process called oxidative stress. Oxidative stress can trigger a number of potentially damaging biochemical reactions.

Antioxidants

It is natural for the body to produce free radicals during cellular metabolism. However, during non-menstruating times, the body also produces natural antioxidants that can counter the effect of free radicals by contributing an electron to free radicals, thereby reducing their reactivity. Antioxidants have the uniqueness of not becoming free radicals themselves even though they contribute electrons to other free radicals.

Oxidative stress during menstruation

The balance between oxidants and antioxidants can be disrupted by an increase in free radicals or a reduction of anti-oxidative substances. In the case of menstruation, both these events occur simultaneously, with the chances of the body going into oxidative stress being high.

During menstruation, the lining of the uterus, called endometrium, breaks down and sheds. Endometrial breakdown and repair are associated with overt inflammation and an influx of inflammatory cells, including neutrophils (granulocyte)[4] and macrophages[5,6]. This indicates an increase in the production of toxic oxygen radicals at the time of menstruation.

Under non-menstruating circumstances, the hormone estrogen plays an important role in neutralizing toxic oxygen radicals. All estrogens have a chemical structure similar to phenolic compounds. This chemical structure makes them capable of offering hydrogen from their phenol-hydroxyl ring. Therefore, they possess reactive oxygen species (ROS)-scavenging, chain-breaking, antioxidant activity. [7, 8] However, during menstruation, estrogen is at an all-time low. In addition, the loss of blood results in the loss of RBCs (red blood cells), which are also known to act as antioxidants that protect the target cells from reactive oxygen species. [9]

Free radicals have been considered as initiators of damage in almost every cellular component. In the female reproductive system, free radicals play various significant roles in the uterine environment, oocyte maturation, ovulation, and corpus luteum function and regression. Studies reveal increased oxidative stress and decreased antioxidants as one of the important contributing factors in the pathogenesis of primary dysmenorrhea (period pain)[10]. Studies also indicate that oxidative stress is known to affect both natural and assisted fertility. Treating infertility due to oxidative stress involves strategies that include identifying the source of excessive generation of ROS, treating the primary cause, and in-vitro and in-vivo supplementation of antioxidants.[11]

Countering oxidative stress during menstruation

When the natural antioxidants in the body are reduced, there is a need to supply antioxidants through dietary intake. Micronutrients in the diet such as vitamins A, C, and E, as well as antioxidant enzymes, are known to neutralize oxygen free radicals and inhibit oxidative stress. Studies indicate that menstruating females should be supplemented with natural antioxidants like vitamin E, vitamin C, and β- carotenoids, which would be extremely useful and may be helpful in combating primary dysmenorrhea[10].

With this background information, when we look at the most common food prescribed by Indian women during menarche and subsequent menstrual periods, we will gain a clearer understanding of how it could prevent menstrual problems, iron-deficiency anemia, and also fertility issues.

1. **Sesame seeds** - Sesame seeds contain sesamol and sesaminol compounds, which are phenolic antioxidants. Together, these compounds help stave off harmful free radicals from the human body. Studies indicate that blood loss of 40 ml[12] during menstruation yields an

average loss of 1.6 mg of iron.[13] Consumption of 100 grams of sesame seeds supplies iron (14.55 mg, 182% RDA),[14] folic acid (97 µg, 25% RDA), calcium (975 mg, 98% RDA), and smaller amounts of vitamin A (9IU), vitamin E (0.25 mg), and carotene-ß (5 µg).[15] Sesame also contains a significant amount of magnesium (351 mg, 88% RDA), which is known to prevent menstrual cramps, dysmenorrhea, and symptoms of PMS, according to several studies.[16, 17]

2. **Jaggery & Dry Coconut** – This combination is almost a must for girls who have just started menstruating. This is likely due to its role in triggering the salivary glands. I realized this during one of my visits to a farmer's house for lunch, where the host served jaggery and dry coconut as an appetizer before the main course. The reason told was that this combination initiates saliva secretion to aid digestion. Put a piece of dry coconut and jaggery in your mouth and experience how it activates the salivary glands. So, the question is about the role of saliva and why it is important during menstruation.

   Human saliva is rich in antioxidant compounds. Salivary antioxidants can be classified in three groups, according to their function: preventive antioxidants, which are those which inhibit the production of free radicals; sweeping antioxidants, which eliminate free radicals in order to inhibit the starting and spreading of cell damage; and thirdly, enzymes such as proteases, transferase, lipases, etc., which repair the damage caused in the tissues.[18] Thus, activating the salivary glands during menstruation helps to combat oxidative stress through the antioxidant properties of saliva.

3. **Urad Dal** – Black gram (vigna mungo) or urad dal is also given to girls during menarche. An important role of urad dal could be the prevention of infertility through its micronutrient value. Studies indicate that women who struggle to conceive have lower than recommended levels of certain micronutrients. For example, insufficient vitamin B12 levels have been reported in more than half of infertile women[19]. Other studies have also found associations between vitamin B12 deficiency and female subfertility.[20,21] Women who are infertile appear to have lower vitamin B6 levels than fertile women. [22]

   Urad dal is an excellent source of B-complex vitamins, such as vitamin B6 - 22%, Thiamin - 23%, Pantothenic acid - 18%, Riboflavin - 20%, and Niacin - 9% of daily recommended values. At 216 μg or 54% of daily values per 100 g, folates are plentiful in black gram. Studies indicate that regular use of multivitamins containing folic acid decreases the risk of ovulatory infertility[23], and a diet high in synthetic folic acid reduces the risk of anovulatory cycles[24] among women with no history of infertility.

   Urad dal is also rich in iron at 7.57 mg or 95% of RDI. Other minerals in ample quantities in these beans are calcium - 14%, copper - 109%, magnesium - 67%, zinc - 30%, and phosphorus - 54% of daily values. They are also rich in potassium—983 mg (21%) per 100 g—nearly 1.5 times more than in chickpeas. Potassium is known to inhibit free radical formation and ROS.[25]

4. **Khichidi** – The main meal recommended during menarche and subsequent menstrual periods is khichidi/

khichiri, a preparation that contains an equal quantity of rice and mũng lentils (vigna radiata). Traditionally, it is instructed to not add salt to khichidi prepared for menstruating girls. Studies indicate that dietary salt causes an increase in oxidative stress.[26]

Mũng lentils are also rich in folates - 625 µg (156% RDA) and other B-complex vitamins. While dry mũng beans hold 4.8 mg or 8% of the daily value of vitamin C, sprouts carry many times more of this vitamin. Vitamin C is a water-soluble antioxidant that helps in boosting immunity and fighting against the oxygen-induced free radicals in the human body. Mũng lentils also contain 6.74 mg iron, which is 84% of the recommended dietary allowance.

5. **Turmeric water for consumption** – A pinch of turmeric powder mixed in water is consumed as a very important part of menarche rituals. Turmeric is famous for its anti-inflammatory and anti-bacterial properties. The main component in turmeric is curcumin, which is known to be an antioxidant. As an antioxidant, turmeric extracts can scavenge free radicals, increase antioxidant enzymes, and inhibit lipid peroxidation.[27]

Restrictions on touching menstruating women

One of the most seemingly discriminatory practices during menstruation pertains to that of not touching menstruating girls/women. As we see during the menarche rituals, if due to some reason, the menstruating girl comes in physical contact with others, then it is necessary for the person(s) who touched her to take a bath.

When we fail to see the science behind this practice, it is but natural that it would seem like discrimination. Let us explore with an open mind and scientific inquiry as to what might be the reason behind this practice. We already know that oxidative stress during menstruation results in the production of more positively charged atoms/ions (cations). Oxidative stress also occurs during ovulation, but the rise of estrogen, which acts as an antioxidant, balances this effect. Whereas during menstruation, estrogen is at its lowest, and as a result, there are excess positively charged ions. This means that there must be a change in the electric potential during ovulation and menstruation, and we should be able to measure it.

Interestingly, there are studies [28,29] which measured the difference in the potential of index fingers of women all through their menstrual cycle. The right index finger showed an increase in positive polarity to several thousands of microvolts between the fourteenth and seventeenth days preceding the onset of the subsequent menses, and also during menses. For nine successive months, this observation was repeated with great accuracy. Menopause, sterility, and male records failed to show such significant peaks. These studies prove that there is a measurable change in electric potential at the time of ovulation and menstruation.

So, what might happen when a menstruating person whose body has more positively charged ions comes in contact with a non-menstruating person whose body has either a neutral charge or a negative charge?

The phenomenon of electron transfer between biological systems or between human beings is relatively new to modern medicine, as it combines the field of biology and quantum physics, which is quantum biology – a subject that is only a decade old. However, a more familiar version of it happens when we experience static electricity. During dry winter seasons, if one were to wear polyester clothing (causing more negative charge to build up) and were to touch a metal (having more positive charge), the electrons jump from the person to the metal. This flow of electrons causes a small electric current, which is sometimes experienced as a mild shock.

The atoms in the positively charged object/body tend to attract electrons in order to neutralize its charge. In the case of menstruating girls/women, they tend to attract electrons from those who touch them. As a result, the person who has touched a menstruating girl experiences a loss of electrons, putting their body at risk of oxidative stress. This is why those who attend to the menstruating girl are required to take a bath before they interact with others. Water in motion (e.g. shower or waterfalls) is said to produce negative ions. Hence, bathing is a good way to regain the loss of electrons by those who are impacted by coming in contact with a menstruating girl/woman. One of the common local practices to prevent menstruating women from affecting young children is to dress the child in flannel. Flannel is an insulator and would thereby prevent the transfer of electrons from the child's body to that of the menstruating woman.

In general, a state where the body has more negative ions is considered to be healthy, while an increase in positive ions indicates a weakened immune system susceptible to disease. Negative ion therapy and negative ionizers are recent inventions aimed at disinfecting spaces to counter infection and disease.[30] Menstruation is a time when the body is naturally in a state where there is a loss of electrons and thereby an increased positive charge. Many of the cultural practices, therefore, aim to expose the menstruating girl to sufficient negative ions to balance this effect, while protecting those who come in contact with her.

Use of turmeric & slaked lime solution

When turmeric is mixed with slaked lime, the resulting red solution is alkaline in nature. The process of mixing slaked lime with turmeric powder increases the water solubility of curcumin through salt formation. Alkaline solutions have a large number of free OH^- ions, which tend to bind with any free H^+ ions.[31] The smearing of the four corners of the mat (on which the menstruating girl sits) with turmeric & slaked lime solution is, therefore, meant to act as an invisible shield around the menstruating girl, preventing her positive ions from spreading and at the same time supplying her with just enough negative ions to keep up her immune system.

As per Āyurved, the mat on which she sits should be made of the darbha grass (Eragrostis cynosuroides), which is known to absorb the positive ions emanating from the menstruating girl's body and provide 'earthing' to the person sitting on it by facilitating a flow of electrons from the earth to the human body. Studies indicate that this plant has an extensive property of acting as anticancerous, antimicrobial, antioxidant agents and has the ability to absorb ultraviolet radiation as well.[32, 33]

Preference for menstrual cloth

Traditionally, Indian women used cotton cloth during menstruation because they preferred it and not because of reasons such as inability to afford sanitary napkins or non-availability of such products. Even now, many women in

India prefer cotton cloth to any other commercially available menstrual product. It is necessary to understand why they have such a preference, especially when products such as sanitary napkins and tampons offer extra-long protection and lesser chances of staining.

While the pH of blood is around 7.5 (slightly alkaline), the vaginal pH is typically 3.5 to 4.5 (moderately acidic). The normal vaginal pH is ideal for beneficial bacteria and creates a hostile environment for pathogenic bacteria that cause odor and infection. When the pH of the vagina increases, it favors the growth of pathogenic bacteria and yeast.[34] During menstruation, vaginal pH becomes elevated by menstrual blood, and chances of contracting infections such as bacterial vaginosis become high.[35] Therefore, breathable menstrual products that require to be changed frequently, such as cotton cloth, help to keep the pH levels in check and prevent vaginal infection. On the other hand, menstrual products that contain an impermeable plastic layer, such as sanitary napkins, and/or are highly absorbent, such as tampons, increase the chances of vaginal infections by increasing the vaginal pH by retaining blood for long periods of time.

Explanations as per native knowledge systems

One might wonder if our ancestors knew enough about these seemingly complex mechanics of menstruation in order to come up with cultural practices to counter it. As I've stated in the introductory chapter, science is one; the variations are only in the depth of understanding. Indigenous sciences knew the mechanisms of menstruation through the knowledge of the subtle anatomy, which can explain, in a simple way, the underlying cause of all the variations seen at the atomic and cellular level.

Prāṇa during menstruation

Some of the answers can be found through an understanding of Prāṇa Vidyā, the science of prāṇa. Prāṇa is the vital life force in a living system. It is not oxygen or air or breath, but rather the life energy that keeps a living being alive. Death occurs when prāṇa leaves the body. The Japanese call it Ki and the Chinese call it Qi or Chi. All oriental sciences understood the way this life force functions and changes as we go through different phases such as menstruation.

In Taoism and Tantra, it is understood that prāṇa is most concentrated in the human seed (sperm and egg), although it circulates throughout the body. As a result, prāṇa is depleted in men by the release of semen, while in women, loss of prāṇa occurs during menstruation and childbirth. The resulting exhaustion and drop in energy levels during menstruation are owing to this loss of prāṇa. Oxygen contains prāṇa. As the body loses prāṇa during menstruation, there is a consequent loss in electrons from the oxygen atom, resulting in an ionic imbalance in the woman's body, causing the atoms in her body to seek electrons from nearby atoms. In the native language, this is explained as a menstruating woman tending to absorb prāṇa from those around her.

Understanding food as per Āyurved

It is interesting to explore how Āyurved's ancient knowledge system was able to identify types of food that would act as antioxidants and provide necessary micronutrition, especially without the calorific and nutritional value information that a modern-day nutritionist would depend on.

One of the classifications of food in Āyurved is based on rasa (taste) and how each rasa has a predominance of particular elements of pañcamahābhūta and thereby exerts a specific effect on the tridoṣa. An overview of the classification of food based on the six types of rasa is given below. A more detailed explanation is provided in the section on Notes titled 'Ṣat Rasa: The Six Tastes'.

Table 1: Ṣat Rasa: **The Six Tastes**

Rasa (taste)	Pañcamahābhūta	Doṣa Subdued	Examples
Madhura (Sweet)	pṛthvi (earth) & āpā (water)	vāta, pitta	ghee (clarified butter), milk, red rice, urad dal (black gram), mūng dal (green gram)
Amla (Sour/ Acid)	pṛthvi (earth) & agni (fire)	vāta	gooseberry, curd, lime, citron, vinegar
Lavana (Saline)	āpā (water) & agni (fire)	vāta	salt, seaweed
Kaṭuka (Pungent)	agni (fire) & vāyu (air)	kapha	pepper, radish, garlic, ginger
Tikta (Bitter)	vāyu (air) & ākāśa (ether)	pitta, kapha	turmeric, neem, bitter gourd
Kashāya (Astringent)	pṛthvi (earth) & vāyu (air)	pitta, kapha	methi (fenugreek), cherry, amaranth

As per the classification of food in Āyurved based on rasa, most of the food prescribed during menarche and subsequent monthly menstruation are of madhura rasa, which plays a role in preventing aggravation of vāta doṣa and pitta doṣa, which are predominant during menstruation.

Dr. Jayashree Nataraj, an Āyurved physician and expert, says, "Āyurved is the only science which speaks of the medicinal value of food, in terms of its effect on doṣa and dhātu." According to Dr. Jayashree, Āyurved also classifies food as Bṛṃhaṇa, Gharṣaṇa, Balya, and Rasāyana, as given below, indicating its special therapeutic value:

- **Bṛṃhaṇa** – food which increases the bulk of the body. This type of food works mainly to increase the māṃsa dhātu (muscle tissue) and not the meda dhātu (fat, adipose tissue). Examples: kharjūra (dates), drakśi (raisin), mudga (mūng/green gram), māṣa (urad/black gram), kuṣmāṇḍa (white pumpkin), tila (sesame), ghee, and milk. These are weight promoters and growth promoters. Food which is of the bṛṃhaṇa category is to be taken soon after menarche, for the first 3-4 months only, to help in the development of the young girl's body.
- **Gharṣaṇa** – food which helps in reducing weight. This type of food works mainly to reduce the meda dhātu (adipose tissue) and does not reduce other dhātus.
- **Balya** – food which increases the overall energy levels or strength (bala) of the body belongs to this category. Food prescribed during menarche is both balya and bṛṃhaṇa in its action.
- **Rasāyana** – food that has rasāyana properties are referred to as sarva dhatu vardhaka, meaning it causes

qualitative, quantitative, and functional enhancement of all dhātus (and also the doṣas as well as the mind). Food such as ghee, milk, jaggery, and all the dry fruits prescribed during menarche have rasāyana properties.

Based on the above knowledge, the type of food prescribed during and soon after menarche can be understood more holistically. According to Suśruta Saṃhita text[36], the properties of each of the food articles (used in menarche practices) are described as below:

- **Urad** – Urad dal/black gram is known as the māṣa pulse in Āyurved texts. It has a sweet taste (madhura rasa), is heavy and pleasant, laxative, diuretic, and demulcent. It subdues vāta and increases kapha.
- **Sesame** – Sesame seeds and oil are very highly recommended in Āyurved texts for various purposes. Also referred to as tila/tilam, it has a taste blended of the sweet and the bitter with a shade of the astringent. It is astringent, heat-making, and generates pitta. It is sweet of digestion, demulcent, acts as a tonic, and subdues the deranged vāta. Of all the different varieties of sesamum, the black species is the best with respect to efficacy. Sesame balances vāta and kapha doṣa and slightly increases pitta (which is why it should not be had in large quantity).
- **Mūng** – Mūng bean/green gram is known as the mudga pulse in Āyurved texts. It is considered as one of the best varieties of pulses since, unlike the other pulses, it does not cause distention of the abdomen caused by gas/air in the organism (tympanites or adhmāna).[36]

- **Rice and Pulses** – Rice boiled and cooked with ghee (clarified butter) and any kind of pulse forms a rich and heavy food which helps to build up new tissues; it imparts strength and rotundity to the body. A soup made of any sort of fried pulse (such as the mudga) without its husks is light and wholesome. Mudga soup subdues kapha and is appetizing and agreeable. It forms the most wholesome diet to persons whose systems have been cleansed with the aid of purgative and emetic remedies. Khichidi made of rice (Āyurved recommends red śāli rice) and split mūng lentils is a gluten-free wholesome meal recommended by Āyurved as a natural cleanser that is easy to digest, thereby preventing over-taxing of the digestive system while the body is busy with menstruation. It prevents aggravation of the doṣas, provides the necessary nutrient intake, and is gentle on the system. According to Dr. Sunil V. Joshi, in his book Ayurveda and Panchakarma, khichidi also liquefies āmā (body toxins) during the second stage of digestion, while the dietary fiber in split mūng beans (16.3 g – 43% RDA) helps to ease the movement of these toxins through the gastrointestinal tract and out of the body.

Therefore, the food prescribed in traditional menarche rituals combines the action of bṛṃhaṇa, balya, and rasāyana, while at the same time preventing aggravation of vāta and pitta, and aiding the elimination of toxins (āmā). This knowledge contained in Āyurved is likely to have been understood by different communities, customized based on availability in their region, and accordingly prescribed to girls who attained menarche.

Impact of menarche rituals

According to a study published in the British Medical Journal (BMJ), titled "Initiation rites at menarche and self-reported dysmenorrhea among indigenous women of the Colombian Amazon: a cross-sectional study" by Zuluaga et al[37]., seven indigenous communities belonging to the Tukano language group were studied. The results show that women not completing the rites were more likely to report dysmenorrhea than those who did so ($p=0.01$); women who completed less than the full complement of rites had a higher risk than those who completed all rites; those who did not complete all initiation rites reported increased severity of dysmenorrhea ($p=0.00014$).

In several Indian homes, menarche rituals and celebrations last for the entire follicular phase of 16 days, starting from the onset of menstruation and ending with ovulation. The importance of these rituals has definitely been overlooked in the modern world. But wise women in India believe that the practices followed during menarche rituals are responsible for maintaining regularity of the monthly cycle, ensuring ovulation, preventing dysmenorrhea (period pain), and even infertility, for the rest of the girl's menstrual years.

As menstrual researchers busy themselves with studies on menstrual products and menstrual hygiene management, areas of true value such as the impact of free radicals and oxidative stress during menstruation, electron transfer during menstruation, the role of specific food as antioxidants for menstruating women, or even the effect of a positive attitude on menstrual health are neither recognized nor studied. Most of the existing studies on menarche and cultural practices are descriptive and offer no scientific understanding of the subject. An entire new field of research is waiting to emerge from a deeper understanding of menarche rituals and their impact on menstrual and reproductive health.

References for Chapter 1

1. Bird, C., Burgess, N. The hippocampus and memory: insights from spatial processing. Nat Rev Neurosci 9, 182–194 (2008)
2. Taittiriya Upanishad
3. Clapp M, Aurora N, Herrera L, Bhatia M, Wilen E, Wakefield S. Gut microbiota's effect on mental health: The gut-brain axis. Clin Pract. 2017;7(4):987. Published 2017 Sep 15.
4. Neutrophils are types of White Blood Cells (WBCs) or granulocyte that protects the body from infections.
5. Macrophages work as innate immune cells through phagocytosis and sterilization of foreign substances such as bacteria, and play a central role in defending the host from infection
6. Garry, R., Hart, R., Karthigasu, K. A. & Burke, C. A re-appraisal of the morphological changes within the endometrium during menstruation: a hysteroscopic, histological and scanning electron microscopic study. Hum Reprod 24, 1393–1401, 2009
7. Sugioka K, Shimosegawa Y, Nakano M. Estrogens as natural antioxidants of membrane phospholipid peroxidation. FEBS Lett 1987; 210: 37–9
8. Moosman B, Behl C. The antioxidant neuroprotective effects of estrogens and phenolic compounds are independent from their estrogenic properties. J Neurosci 1999; 96: 8867–72
9. Pandey, K. B., & Rizvi, S. I. (2010). Markers of oxidative stress in erythrocytes and plasma during aging in humans. Oxidative medicine and cellular longevity, 3(1), 2–12.

10. S.Venkata Rao, Ravi Kiran.V.S, M. Vijaysree. Oxidative stress and antioxidant status in primary dysmenorrhea. Journal of Clinical and Diagnostic Research. 2011 June, Vol-5(3): 509-511)
11. A. Agarwal, S.S. Allamaneni. Role of free radicals in female reproductive diseases and assisted reproduction. Reprod. Biomed. Online, 9 (3) (2004 Jan 1), pp. 338-347
12. Blood loss around menstruation is said to be between 30ml to 80ml. When it exceeds 80ml, it is considered as heavy menstrual bleeding.
13. Jacob A Butler E Blanche M. Menstrual blood loss in iron deficiency anemia. Lancet. 1965; 407:1102–1107.
14. RDA is Recommended Dietary Allowance
15. The nutritional values mentioned for all the edibles are as per USDA National Nutrient data base
16. Fontana-Klaiber H, Hogg B. Therapeutische Wirkung von Magnesium bei Dysmenorrhöe [Therapeutic effects of magnesium in dysmenorrhea]. Schweiz Rundsch Med Prax. 1990;79(16):491-494.
17. Seifert, B., Wagler, P., Dartsch, S., Schmidt, U., & Nieder, J. (1989). Magnesium--a new therapeutic alternative in primary dysmenorrhea. Zentralblatt fur Gynakologie, 111(11), 755-760.
18. Ivan Minic. Antioxidant Role of Saliva. Journal of Otolaryngology: Research. 2019; 2(1):124
19. La Vecchia I, Paffoni A, Castiglioni M, et al. Folate, homocysteine and selected vitamins and minerals status in infertile women. Eur J Contracept Reprod Health Care. 2017;22:70–75.

20. Bennett M. Vitamin B12 deficiency, infertility and recurrent fetal loss. J Reprod Med. 2001;46:209–212.
21. El-Nemr A, Sabatini L, Wilson C, Lower AM, Al-Shawaf T, Grudzinskas JG. Vitamin B12 deficiency and IVF. J Obstet Gynaecol. 1998;18:192–193.
22. Grajecki D, Zyriax B-C, Buhling K. The effect of micronutrient supplements on female fertility: a systematic review. Arch Gynecol Obstet. 2012;285:1463–1471.
23. Chavarro JE, Rich-Edwards JW, Rosner BA, Willett WC. Use of multivitamins, intake of B vitamins, and risk of ovulatory infertility. Fertil Steril. 2008;89:668–676.
24. Gaskins AJ, Mumford SL, Chavarro JE, et al. The impact of dietary folate intake on reproductive function in premenopausal women: a prospective cohort study. PLoS One. 2012;7:e46276.
25. McCabe RD, Bakarich MA, Srivastava Kumud, Young, DB. Potassium inhibits free radical formation. https://www.ahajournals.org/doi/pdf/10.1161/01.HYP.24.1.77
26. Kitiyakara C, Chabrashvili T, Chen Y, Blau J, Karber A, Aslam S, Welch WJ, Wilcox CS. Salt intake, oxidative stress, and renal expression of NADPH oxidase and superoxide dismutase. J Am Soc Nephrol 2003 Nov; 14(11):2775-82.
27. Cohly H. H, Taylor A, Angel M. F, Salahudeen A. K. Effect of turmeric, turmerin and curcumin on H2O2-induced renal epithelial (LLC-PK1) cell injury. Free Radic Biol Med. 1998;24:49–54.
28. Barton, Dorothy S. Electric Correlates of The Menstrual Cycle in Women. Yale Journal of Biology and Medicine, 1940.
29. Burr H.S., Musselman L.K. Bio-electric phenomena associated with menstruation. Yale Journal of Biology and Medicine, 1936

30. McDowell. Air inonizers wipe out hospital infections. www.newscientist.com, 3 Jan 2003
31. Ravindran P.N, Babu K.N, Sivaraman, K. Turmeric: The genus Curcuma, 2007
32. M. Barath, J. Aravind, R. Sivasamy. Investigation of Antimicrobial activity and Chemical Constituents of Eragrostis cynosuroides by GC-MS. Research J. Pharm. and Tech. 9(3): Mar., 2016; Page 267-271.
33. Sakhalkar, Sachin, Kambale, Naina. Study of Biological activity of Eragrostis cynosuroides (B.A.) based on Ayurveda's Literature. Indian Journal of Applied Research. Volume : 4 | Issue : 4 | Apr 2014 | ISSN - 2249-555X
34. Dr. Seibel, Machelle. Menstruation, infection and the pH connection. Feb 17, 2010. www.businesswire.com
35. Wagner, Ottesen. Vaginal physiology during menstruation. Annals of internal medicine, 1982 Jun;96(6 Pt 2):921-3.
36. Kaviraj Kunja Lal Bhishagratna, An English Translation of Sushrutha Samhita, Vol 1 – Suthrasthanam, 1907
37. Zuluaga G, Andersson N Initiation rites at menarche and self-reported dysmenorrhoea among indigenous women of the Colombian Amazon: a cross-sectional study BMJ Open 2013;3:e002012.
38. Swami Niranjanananda Saraswati. Prana Pranayama Prana Vidya. 1994
39. Vaidya Atreya Smith. Prana: The Secret of Yogic Healing. 1993
40. Yogi Ramacharaka. The Science of Psychic Healing, 1906

CHAPTER 2

DECODING MENSTRUAL PRACTICES THROUGH ĀYURVED

मासन्निष्पिच्छदाहार्ति पंचरात्रानुबन्धि च |
नैवातिबह नात्यल्पमार्तवं शुद्दमादिशेत् ||
गुंजाफलसवर्णं च पद्मालक्तकसन्निभम्
इन्द्रगोपसंकाशमार्तवं शुद्दमादिशेत् ||

- (च. चि. - ३०)

māsaniṣpicchadāhārti pañcarātrānubandhi ca
naivātibaha nātyalpamārtavaṃ śuddhamādiśet
guñjāphalasavarṇam ca padmālaktakasannibham
indragopasankāśamārtavaṃ śuddhamādiśet

– (Caraka Saṃhita - 30)

Thousands of years ago, seers of Āyurved defined a healthy menstrual discharge very clearly. According to the above verses from Caraka Saṃhita, ārtava (menstrual flow) is said to be healthy if it has the following features: niṣpiccha – free from sliminess of discharge; dāhārti – (free from) burning sensation and pain; pañcarātrānubandhi – lasts for five nights; na ati bahu na aplam – flow is neither too heavy nor too scanty; guñjā phala sa varṇam – the color of menstrual discharge is like the gunja fruit (rosary pea/abrus precatorius); padma alaktata sannibham – or (the color) is similar to the lotus or Indragopa insect (trombidium).

शशासृक्प्रतिमं यत् तु यद्वा लाक्षारसोपमम् ।
तदार्तवं प्रशंसन्ति यद् वासो न विरंजयेत् ॥

- (सु. शा. - २/१७)

śaśāsrukpratimam yat tu yadvā lākṣārasopamam
tadārtavam praśamsanti yad vāso na viramjayet

– (Suśruta Saṃhita)

Again, in the verses of Suśruta Saṃhita given above, healthy menstrual discharge is described as the catamenial blood[1] (ārtava), which is red like the blood of a hare (śaśāsrukpratimam), or the washings of shellac[2] (lākṣārasopamam), and leaves no stains on clothes (which may be washed off by simply soaking them in water) (vāso na viramjayet).

While most advertisements on menstrual products today treat menstrual stain as the worst thing possible, in Āyurved, a stain is an important indication of how healthy a period is. By putting a drop of menstrual blood on a cotton cloth, allowing it to dry, washing it with water, and observing if it leaves a stain or not, women should be able to get an indication of the state of their menstrual health. This might also be one of the reasons why traditionally, in Indian society, women preferred using cotton cloth to absorb menstrual flow.

Āyurved does not consider period pain, irregular menstruation, or changing bleeding patterns every month as normal, regardless of how common it might have become. Each time the period varies, it is an important indication of knowing the imbalances in the body and taking measures to correct it. Being able to decode menstrual health through observation of the color, texture, quantity, and flow of menstrual blood can be a fantastic way to detect problems early on and prevent it from snowballing into a disease. This is what knowledge of Āyurved can do for menstruating women.

Tridoṣa

What sets Āyurved apart from allopathy (Western medicine) is its fine understanding of the sūkṣma śarīra (subtle body) in addition to the sthūla śarīra (gross body). Therefore, in addition to the understanding of organs, tissues, cells, and hormones, Āyurved recognizes three types of subtle internal forces that control all functions within the body. These are the three internal bodily forces called the tri-doṣas. Tri refers to the number three, and doṣa literally means 'fault' or that which causes things to spoil. If the three doṣas (vāta, pitta, kapha) are not in a state of equilibrium, disease is said to arise. It is called a doṣa, since both excess and lack can cause an imbalance, resulting in disease. Every individual has a specific prakṛti (body constitution) arising from the combination of the three doṣas, and accordingly, it influences individual health and personality. In women, it also influences menstruation and the quality of menstrual blood.

Dhātu

Āyurved describes seven tissue layers called dhātu, starting with rasa (chyle). The lymph chyle or rasa, formed as a result of digestion, courses through the body and contains the subtle elements which build the different tissues (dhātu) of the human organism. Under the influence of metabolic heat (pitta), rasa is progressively transformed into rakta (blood), māṃsa (flesh), medas (fat), asthi (bone), majjā (marrow), and śukra (semen/ovum), which are the seven dhātu.[3]

Rasa is successively transformed into each of the six remaining dhātu and continues in the form of each dhātu for the period of three thousand and fifteen kālā, which is five days according to our modern computation. Thus, the rasa is converted into semen in men, or ovum in women, in the course of a month. Menstrual blood is considered as a by-product of the rasa dhātu. Hence, the essence of the food we consume greatly influences the quality of menstrual blood. More information about the formation of dhātu is provided in the section of Notes titled 'Dhātu'.

Rajaswala Paricaryā/menstrual regime

Āyurved texts list several dos and don'ts during menstruation which are termed Rajaswala Paricaryā and refers to the regime prescribed for menstruating women. According to Suśruta Saṃhitā[4], practices prescribed during menstruation include avoiding sexual intercourse, excessive talking, excessive laughing, exposure to loud noise, crying, applying collyrium[5] to the eyes, sleeping during the day, combing the hair, paring the nails, taking bath, oil massage, anointing the body (with sandalwood paste, etc.), and avoiding fatiguing work.

At first glance, these practices may seem unreasonable, and it is not hard to imagine why some women might consider these as oppressive. But if we can keep an open mind and approach with genuine curiosity, we will arrive at many interesting answers which will forever change the way we perceive and, more importantly, experience menstruation.

As a subject, Āyurved is very vast, and it is difficult to grasp all of it without a formal course. However, for our purpose, we will touch upon those aspects which are related to menstruation. I often find that the best way to understand Āyurved is in a context. In this case, the context of Rajaswala Paricaryā presents a good opportunity to understand both Āyurved and menstrual practices in a new light. I recommended the book Ayurvedic Healing for Women, by Atreya[6], especially for those who are new to Āyurved and would like to gain insights into reproductive health as per Āyurved. In the following paragraphs, the three doṣas, their function, and menstrual practices associated with them are explained, as inferred from Suśruta Saṃhitā and Caraka Saṃhitā.

The tridoṣa of Vāyu (also called vāta or vāt), Pitta (also called pittam or pith), and Kapha (also called śleṣma or kapham or kaph) respectively occupy the lower, middle, and upper portions of the body. The terms vāta, pitta, and śleṣma (kapha) are respectively derived from the roots 'va', to move or smell, 'tāpā', to burn or to heat, and 'śliṣā', to embrace. From this, it should be inferred that motion and smell are the natural attributes of vāta; heat and burning are those of pitta; union and integration are those of kapha. The vāyu or vāta is a self-originated principle in the human organism. The pitta owes its origin to the bodily heat (āgneya), while the origin of kapha is ascribed to the presence of watery (saumya) principle in the body.

Vāta doṣa

Vāta doṣa has the qualities of śīta (coolness), rūkṣatā (roughness), laghu (lightness), vaiśadya (non-slimy), gati (movement), and anavasthitatva (instability).[7] It is the principal nerve force within the body; consequently, all nervous disorders are due to an imbalanced vāta. Vāta organizes all functions and movements within the body—circulation, respiration, muscular movement, motor function, the five sense organs, excretion, menstruation, lactation, and even birthing. An imbalanced vāta doṣa can impair the functioning of these activities.

Bones and the skeletal system are also influenced by the state of vāta; this means that excessive vāta can cause dryness in the bones and make them brittle. Vāta also influences the endocrine system and consequently the play of hormones, especially during menstruation. Stress directly impacts vāta and the nervous system, causing problems like irregular menstrual cycles.

The primary seat of vāta is the intestinal tract and the rectum. When in balance, it maintains a state of equilibrium between the doṣas and dhātus. A disturbance in vāta will manifest itself as digestive disorders such as constipation or gastric problems in the early stages. An impaired vāta is responsible for most diseases, especially menstrual and reproductive disorders.

People with vāta prakṛti[8] might exhibit external qualities such as dry skin and hair, thin/wiry body frame, restlessness or fidgety nature, hurried speech, and an occasional feeling of floating in the air (similar to a jet lag) when vāta doṣa is not in balance. Emotionally, imbalanced vāta will express itself as irritation, anxiousness, mood swings, and a fluctuating personality. When in balance, people with a dominant vāta personality will be creative, intuitive, hard-working, and adaptable, with a love for travel because of their inherent quality of movement.

Vāta doṣa has five subtypes, which are described in the section on Notes titled 'Subtypes of Doṣa'.

Menstruation in vāta prakṛti women

Since vāta is responsible for all movements, the flow of menstrual blood has a dominance of vāta doṣa. The qualities of vāta prakopa (increased vāta) will be seen in a menstruating woman when vāta is in excess. Women with an inherent vāta prakṛti (vāta dominant body constitution) have a greater tendency of menstruating with characteristics of vāta prakopa. However, other women too can experience menses with vāta prakopa during the months when their vāta has been aggravated; for example, after excessive travel or strenuous physical exercise in the days preceding menstruation, or consumption of very cold food during menses. The menstrual discharge with vāta qualities will have the following characteristics based on vāta prakṛti or vāta prakopa.

Table 2: Menstrual Characteristics based on vāta

	Vāta Prakṛti (Normal)	Vāta Prakopa (Problematic)
Color	Slightly darker than normal	Dark brownish blood
Flow	Flow is on the lesser side	Scanty blood flow or only spots
Texture	Thin in consistency	Non-sticky texture
Physical discomfort	Nil	Menstrual cramps and pain in the lower abdomen, constipation, flatulence, pain in the pelvis and thighs, throbbing pain in the calf
Emotional state	No obvious change	Feeling of restlessness, irritation, anxiousness
Menstrual problems most likely for women with dominant vāta doṣa	Irregular menses, especially soon after menarche	Dysmenorrhea (period pain), amenorrhea (delayed or no period), and irregular menses

When in good health, a vāta-prakṛti woman will experience a light period for a short duration, between 2-4 days, free of emotional instability and physical discomfort. If menstruating women observe their physical and emotional state each month, they will be able to identify whether or not they exhibit characteristics of vāta prakopa or are tending toward it. Personally, this observation has helped me bring awareness to my health each month, especially when at times the necessities of a hectic work schedule leave little room for self-care. Early identification can play an important role in understanding the cause of menstrual discomfort and making changes in diet and lifestyle practices to bring one's health back to normalcy.

Menstrual regime to prevent vāta prakopa

Since vāta is naturally dominant during the course of menstruation, most of the menstrual practices mentioned in Āyurved pertain to preventing a state of vāta prakopa, given that vāta is more susceptible to aggravation during menstruation.

Avoiding strong emotions - Strong emotions that disturb the nervous system such as excessive laughter, crying, loud noise, and even excessive talking can aggravate vāta, especially in a menstruating woman. These actions may seem harmless on a non-menstruating day when we are able to come back to normalcy after a while. But at the time of menstruation, the natural dominance of vāta makes the nervous system extra sensitive, and such harmless acts could also trigger a disturbance in the menstrual flow.

It is not uncommon that women who have been through a sudden shock or have undergone periods of prolonged grief can sometimes even miss a period. The study by Hannoun AB, et al. on the "Effects of war on the menstrual cycle"[9] showed that acute stressful conditions like that of a war resulted in menstrual abnormalities in 10%-35% of the women.

Avoid combing hair and paring nails - When in stress, we might observe that hair fall is more than usual. Stress results in the aggravation of vāta. The dominance of vāta during menstruation will create a similar situation as stress, making hair brittle and more likely to fall. Similarly, nakhābheda (cracking of nails) is a condition that occurs when vāta is imbalanced. As per Āyurved, hair and nails are products of the asthi (bone) dhātu. Therefore, anything that affects the asthi dhātu could also affect hair and nails.

Avoid fatiguing work - Excessive physical exercise or fatiguing work during menstruation can cause bone-related injuries more easily, since an aggravated vāta makes the bones brittle. There is more on this subject in the chapter titled 'Sports and Menstruation: Why It Doesn't Have to be Painful'.

Other practices - While most of the above practices are meant to prevent the increase of vāta, certain practices serve the opposite purpose. For example, sleeping during the day, anointing the body, and undergoing an oil massage—these practices have the effect of reducing vāta and are normally recommended for balancing vāta after heavy exercise or travel. However, for menstruation to occur as it should, the naturally dominant vāta during menstruation should not be tampered with, and therefore, such practices are also recommended to be avoided, as per Āyurved.

Pitta doṣa

Pitta has the qualities of uṣṇa (heat), tīkṣṇa sharpness), dravatva (liquidity), sneha (unctuousness/oily), visra gandha (smells like fish), kaṭu & amla (pungent and sour) taste, and saratva (fluidity)[7]. Pitta has the predominance of agni (fire), giving it the property of transformation. Pitta controls all transformative activities within the body such as digestion, metabolism, and ovulation. Therefore, an imbalanced pitta doṣa can result in excessive agni, which burns up food too quickly, preventing the absorption of essential nutrients, or manda (dull) agni, which could slow down digestion and metabolism. The insufficient absorption of nutrients, which is more likely to happen for those with high pitta, could result in anemia. Pitta also influences eyesight, and aggravated pitta[10] can impact vision. Pitta governs the health of the skin and liver and results in skin problems when aggravated. Internally, pitta is present as digestive acids and bile. The primary seat of pitta is the liver and spleen, the heart, the pupils of the eye, the skin, and the small intestines. During menstruation, pitta is also dominant since blood has pitta properties. Factors that derange the pitta also vitiate the blood.

People with pitta prakṛti might exhibit external qualities such as acne, sensitive skin and skin rashes, inflammation, premature graying of hair, workaholic tendencies, an overheated body, hunger, thirst, frequent digestion imbalances, and spells of fainting when pitta is imbalanced. Emotionally, excessive pitta will express itself as anger, extreme short temper, frustration, jealously, judgmental nature, and a controlling personality. However, when in balance, people with a dominant pitta personality will have leadership qualities, strong intellect, will be passionate, and have good communication skills. Their body type is generally athletic, and they do not put on weight easily. Pitta doṣa has five subtypes, which are described in the section on Notes titled 'Subtypes of Doṣa'.

Menstruation in pitta prakṛti women

The qualities of pitta prakopa (increased pitta) will be seen in a menstruating woman when pitta is high. Women with an inherent pitta prakṛti (pitta dominant body constitution) have a greater tendency of menstruating with characteristics of pitta prakopa. However, other women too can experience menses with pitta prakopa during the months when their pitta has been aggravated; for example, due to excessive consumption of spicy, non-vegetarian, or heat-generating food just before or during menstruation. The menstrual discharge with pitta qualities will have the following characteristics based on pitta prakṛti or pitta prakopa.

Table 3: Menstrual Characteristics based on Pitta

	Pitta prakṛti (Normal)	Pitta prakopa (Problematic)
Color	Bright red	Bright red
Flow	Flow is slightly more than average	Heavy and hot flow, might have a metallic odor
Texture	Neither too thin nor too sticky	Sometimes has clots
Physical discomfort	Nil	Acne, tenderness of breasts, inflammation, body heat/feverish feeling, headache, diarrhea, soreness, tiredness
Emotional effect	Nil	Irritability, fatigue, anger, and short temper
Menstrual problems most likely for women with dominant pitta doṣa	Nil	Menorrhagia (heavy menstrual bleeding), anemia

When in balance, women of pitta-prakṛti will experience slightly profuse but regular menstruation of average duration between 3 and 5 days. The absence of sudden bouts of anger will be an indication of having balanced pitta. Women can observe their menstrual flow each month for qualities that are indicative of pitta prakopa and take measures to reduce internal heat, especially by including food that is śīta (cooling in nature) and avoiding food that is uṣṇa (heating in nature). When early signs of excessive pitta are identified by observing the menstrual flow and necessary diet and lifestyle modifications are made, it could prevent conditions such as menorrhagia (heavy menstrual bleeding) caused by pitta prakopa.

Menstrual regime to prevent pitta prakopa

Most of the menstrual practices pertaining to food have to do with preventing pitta aggravation. As per Āyurved, food is classified based on its properties of uṣṇa (heating) or śīta (cooling) when consumed. This is different from the external hot or cold sensation of food and refers to how the food behaves after consumption. For example, refrigerated curd, which seems cold, when consumed has the uṣṇa or heating (acidic) property. All non-vegetarian food (including egg), caffeine, alcohol, smoking, and spicy food have the uṣṇa properties, thereby increasing internal heat or pitta (experienced as acidity). Sour food articles like curd or lemon also increase pitta. Even fruits like papaya and oranges are to be avoided during menstruation as it can increase the already dominant pitta during menstruation. In short, partaking of food consisting of pungent, acid, sour, or saline taste, as well as of those whose digestion is followed by a reactionary acidity, will aggravate pitta. The result of consuming such food just before or during menstruation, especially for one who is of a pitta prakṛti, could be excessively hot and heavy bleeding. Details of the categorization of food into six types and the impact of each type on the doṣas is given in the section on Notes titled 'Ṣat Rasa: The Six Tastes'.

Application of collyrium – In tropical regions, there is a traditional practice of applying collyrium or kajal to the inner part of the eyelid. While women largely follow this practice, in several regions with hot climatic conditions, men too use collyrium. Unlike the modern use of it, in ancient societies, it was not just a cosmetic. Traditionally, collyrium was made from medicinal herbs and ghee, which cool the eye and prevent eye-related disorders. When temperatures are high, pitta is high. Since pitta impacts vision, a rise in pitta can affect eyesight. To prevent this, collyrium is used, as it has a cooling effect on pitta. However, during menstruation, pitta is naturally dominant and should not be tampered with. Therefore, the application of collyrium is restricted for menstruating women. (Note that if it is just a cosmetic with no cooling properties, it can probably be used even during menstruation). For similar reasons, using henna (Lawsonia inermis) during menstruation is to be avoided, as henna has cooling properties.

Rules for bathing – In most traditional Indian homes, children are taught to avoid taking bath soon after a meal as it impairs the health. This is because of the understanding that taking a bath after a meal dampens the pitta/digestive acids necessary to digest the food. It is akin to pouring water on a cooking pot that has just begun to gather heat. As a result, the food remains undigested, causing the formation of bodily toxins called āmā, which is said to be the root cause of several diseases.

According to Suśruta Saṃhitā, bathing in extremely cold water in winter tends to enrage the bodily vāyu and the kapha, while bathing in hot water in summer agitates the blood and the pitta. Bathing is not beneficial for fever, diarrhea, earache, tympanites, aversion to food, indigestion, and in the disorders or diseases due to the actions of the deranged vāta. It should also not be taken just after a meal. In the cases where bathing is prohibited, anulepana (anointing the body with scented pastes) is also prohibited.

During menstruation, one should not tamper with the naturally dominant pitta and vāta, and taking a bath is therefore not recommended. Further, being underwater during menstruation has the tendency to temporarily stop the menstrual flow; women can observe this even during a shower.

Traditionally, women are told to keep themselves warm during menstruation, so as to maintain the internal temperature required for the blood flow to happen smoothly. However, for hygiene purposes, rural women have modified some of these practices such as not taking a bath. The modified practice which is very prevalent in South India is to wash one's hair immediately after the start of menstruation and on the last day of menstruation, while a light washing of the body, without pouring water on the head, continues on all other days. During my workshops on menstruation in South India, the seemingly strange practice of washing one's hair on day one and day four of menstruation are among the top questions that women struggle to make sense of.

Kapha doṣa

Kapha doṣa has the qualities of sneha (unctuousness), śīta (cooling), śauklya (whiteness), gaurava (heaviness), madhura (sweetness), sthairya (steadiness), paicchilya (sliminess), and mārtsnya (viscosity). Kapha doṣa is responsible for maintaining the structure and stability of cells within the body and is responsible for providing the base fluid during menstruation.

It is responsible for hydrating the internal cells and systems, lubricating the joints, maintaining immunity, and protecting the tissues. The primary seat of kapha is the stomach, the breast, the throat, the head, and the joints. When in excess, it is released as phlegm.

People with kapha prakṛti might exhibit external qualities such as a tendency to gain weight easily, slow digestion, heaviness, excessive sleep, sedentary habits, and chronic respiratory problems such as asthma or sinusitis when kapha is not in balance. Internally, an imbalance in kapha will express itself as lethargy, laziness, food cravings, feelings of unworthiness, and sadness. However, when in balance, kapha dominant personalities are easy-going people, given their stable temperament. Their heavy body type gives them the qualities of endurance, stamina, and physical strength, making them good at sports like weightlifting and marathons. Kapha prakṛti women are also considered to have the best fertility.

Menstruation in kapha prakṛti women

The qualities of kapha prakopa (increased kapha) will be seen in a menstruating woman when kapha is high. Women with an inherent kapha prakṛti (kapha dominant body constitution) have a greater tendency of menstruating with characteristics of kapha prakopa. However, other women too can experience menses with kapha prakopa during the months when their kapha has been aggravated; for example, when one is suffering from cold and excess phlegm. The menstrual discharge with kapha qualities will have the following characteristics based on kapha prakṛti or kapha prakopa.

Table 4: Menstrual Characteristics as per Kapha

	Kapha prakṛti (Normal)	Kapha prakopa (Problematic)
Color	Not very bright red	Light red color
Flow	Moderate flow	Moderate flow
Texture	Thick and slimy (presence of mucous)	Thick and slimy with clots
Physical discomfort	Moderate heaviness	Water retention and increase in body weight, heaviness, increased sleep. Indigestion, with feelings of nausea, occasional vomiting, and a continuous dull ache
Emotional effect	Laziness	Depression
Menstrual problems most likely for women with dominant kapha doṣa	Nil	Slightly more susceptible to leukorrhea (excessive/ abnormal white discharge) before menstruation. Itching and yeast infections are also more likely

Kapha women have the longest duration of menstrual flow, lasting up to seven days, is regular yet light, and devoid of menstrual discomfort when in balance. Women with a kapha prakṛti sometimes feel a great relief at the onset of menstruation, as the heaviness of kapha gets balanced by the natural dominance of pitta and vāta during menstruation. We can observe this during times when we have a kapha related problem such as the common cold, which relieves itself after menstruation.

Menstrual regime to prevent kapha prakopa

Since kapha doṣa is not predominant during menstruation, there are no menstrual practices that are specific to kapha. In the case of women with dominant kapha prakṛti, care needs to be taken to keep kapha in balance at all times, so that it does not cause menstrual pain and discomfort. Activities that build pitta such as frequent exercise (except during menstruation) and avoiding stale, heavy food will greatly benefit kapha women and ease their menstrual flow.

Please note - A common question among women pertains to why one woman's menstrual flow is different from that of another woman. While modern medicine does not have a clear answer to this, Āyurved can explain the uniqueness of each woman's period with the help of the doṣas. Most individuals are a combination of doṣas such as vāta-pitta, vāta-kapha, pitta-kapha, etc. Consequently, their personalities, and in women, their menstrual discharge, have the characteristics of all the doṣas at play.

Disease causes a temporary condition called vikṛti, which might cause a change in the inherent doṣas, for the duration of the disease. Only a qualified Āyurved practitioner will be able to assess the inherent prakṛti and the temporary vikṛti, and one must not make assumptions by reading books alone. The information provided above is for general purposes only, and one must consult an Āyurved practitioner who is adept at nāḍī parīkṣā or prakṛti parīkṣā, to get a correct assessment of one's doṣa type.

Sexual abstinence during menstruation

Āyurved texts have several regulations regarding sexual intimacy between married couples. It is important to note that

Suśruta Saṃhitā mentions all the above menstrual practices in the context of attempting to conceive a child after menstruation, since days four to 12 of the menstrual cycle (day one being the first day of menstruation) are considered ideal for conceiving a child. When it comes to sexual intercourse, the regulations are not just for women, but also for the woman's husband/partner. In order to conceive a healthy child, the husband is advised to maintain sexual abstinence for one month prior to his wife's next menses, and strictly abstain from sexual intimacy for the first three days of menstruation. In Suśruta Samhita's Cikitsa Sthānam, there is a chapter pertaining to hygiene and prophylactic measures in general. Here, among the many practices for preventing disease among men, it is mentioned that visiting a woman in her menses results in the loss of sight, longevity, and vital power, and it should be accordingly considered as a sinful act.[11]

Suśruta Saṃhitā mentions that sexual intercourse during day one or two of menstruation can shorten the husband's life, and the child, if born, dies immediately or within the first ten days. Sexual intercourse during day three of menstruation can cause the child to be born deformed and short-lived. Whereas, a child born out of intercourse on the fourth day[12] of the menstrual cycle will be healthy and will live long. Other days to attempt to conceive go up to the twelfth day. Once impregnated, the husband is advised to practice sexual abstinence for a month after the twelfth day of his wife's menstrual cycle. The duration of one month's abstinence is likely to be because the rasa (the essence of food consumed) is converted into semen (śukra dhātu) in the course of a month.

The menstrual practices mentioned in Suśruta Saṃhitā ensure that there will not be any doṣa imbalance in the woman's body, as it is assumed that she will be attempting to conceive soon after her menses. Birth of a child was given immense importance in Āyurved texts, and several practices are recommended to ensure that the child born is healthy and not deformed in any way. These practices help to create the ideal womb in which a child can be born.

In today's times, women are unlikely to attempt to conceive every cycle, even if they are not already pregnant. So, the question that arises is whether sexual abstinence during menstruation is still necessary. There are reasons why sexual intercourse during menstruation could negatively impact the menstruating woman and her partner.

Sexual intercourse is prohibited for women during menstruation as it aggravates the nervous system and hence vāta becomes greatly disturbed. Further, the friction caused increases the heat, pitta. A menstruating women's body attempts to make up for the loss of prāṇa by absorbing the prāṇa of those around her (this is explained in terms of ions in the previous chapter). Men lose prāṇa whenever they lose semen. This loss of prāṇa by men is compounded during intercourse with a menstruating woman. Loss of prāṇa in men creates a lack of vitality and strength. This is likely to be the reason why men who have intercourse with menstruating women (and do not compensate for the loss of prāṇa through certain rituals/ practices) are said to have a shorter lifespan, as per Āyurved texts.

Other menstrual practices

Apart from the practices mentioned in Āyurved texts, many others have emerged based on local contexts and the influence of native knowledge systems. Few such practices are explained below.

Avoiding touching of plants or infants during menstruation

I learned something interesting from rural women in a village in Sandur (Bellary district, Karnataka) during my workshop on menstruation. In their culture, when a girl attains menarche, she is given a plant to water and nurture all through her bleeding days. The plant is then closely observed over the next few weeks to see if it withers away or remains unaffected. If it withers away, then the girl is told not to touch plants or infants when she menstruates henceforth. Thus, women do their own experiment to figure out if the practice should apply to the girl or not, rather than having a common rule for all menstruating girls.

To me, this was evidence of a deeper knowledge that not all girls are alike and not all of them can affect plants or others when they menstruate. It is likely that girls who have a dominant vāta or pitta doṣa are more likely to cause withering of a sensitive plant like the tulasī and similarly affect the health of an infant. Tulasī (Ocimum santum) is revered in India because of its abundance of prāṇa and its capacity to increase the prāṇa of those who come in contact with it. When a menstruating woman comes close to, or touches the plant, it is possible that the plant goes into oxidative stress. Studies indicate that oxidative stress can be harmful to plants as well.[13]

Similarly, a new life such as an infant is also a bundle of prāṇa. When menstruating women come in close contact with such prāṇa, their tendency to absorb this vital life force creates a resulting imbalance in the body which loses prāṇa. At the same time, menstruating women are supposed to lose a certain amount of prāṇa, which flows downwards and outwards, whereas coming in contact with a plant like tulasī will cause an upward rise in their prāṇa, thereby disturbing the menstrual flow.

From my own experience as someone who has a pitta prakṛti, I have seen how the tulasī plant struggles to grow if I am around it at the time of menses. This needs to be observed over a period of a few weeks to notice the slow withering away of the plant. Similar experiences have been shared with me by other women as well.

I have also heard women say that by looking at the color and quality of an infant's stool, they can tell whether or not the child has come in contact with a menstruating woman. This could be because diarrhea is caused due to an increase in pitta (and consequent discoloration)[17], which could happen when the infant comes in contact with a menstruating woman.

Avoiding cooking of food

Anyone who is slightly observant will be able to tell the difference in taste when food is prepared from freshly sourced vegetables and when food is prepared from vegetables that are a few days old or refrigerated. What makes this difference in taste possible even though, externally, fresh vegetables might look the same as vegetables kept in cold storage? The differentiating factor is prāṇa. All living things contain prāṇa. When plant food is freshly harvested, it still contains prāṇa and that is what makes it healthy and tasty. As days go by, prāṇa slowly leaves and the food is no longer as healthy or tasty.

Menstruating women have the capacity to absorb prāṇa from anything that contains it. In the case of food, this would affect both the taste and health aspects of the food being prepared. At the same time, the downward coursing apāna (a subtype of vāta responsible for menstrual flow) in menstruating women will be confused by the upward rising prāṇa in fresh plant food. Many women, including me, have observed the reduced taste in food cooked during menstruation even though the recipe is followed perfectly.

In the Hindu way of life, great importance is attached to spiritual practices, and traditionally, almost every household had people who were on a spiritual path. For such persons, food from which the prāṇa has been drained, be it animal flesh, stale plant food, or food touched by a menstruating woman, comes in the way of their spiritual process. This is also one of the reasons why menstruating women have traditionally avoided cooking for the family.

Avoiding silkworm rearing

Another practice that I have come across in some villages where silkworm rearing is a primary occupation is that menstruating women do not enter the rearing house. When the cocoon is still developing, it is very sensitive to temperature changes. The worms also generate heat, which is why rearing houses are kept as cool as possible.

Silkworm rearers will explain that they have seen how the worms die when a menstruating woman enters the room, and hence the practice. However, the opposite, that is, the woman being impacted by the worms, is also possible. During one of my visits to a village in Chamarajanagar district of Karnataka, as part of a pre-screening exercise for menstrual disorders among rural women, I witnessed something unusual. Some of the women who I interviewed were in their early or late thirties but had already reached menopause. The health worker who accompanied me said that this is a strange phenomenon that she has seen in this village and that it was more predominant especially one generation earlier. As I began entering the homes to interview the women, I noticed that some of them were rearing silkworms in vertical baskets, inside the house. Usually, there is a separate rearing room, but these families were so poor that they did not have space for a separate room, and they slept beside the worm baskets. These were older women who had reached menopause when in their thirties and still practiced silkworm rearing. The younger generation did other jobs, and the practice of rearing silkworms inside their homes was discontinued.

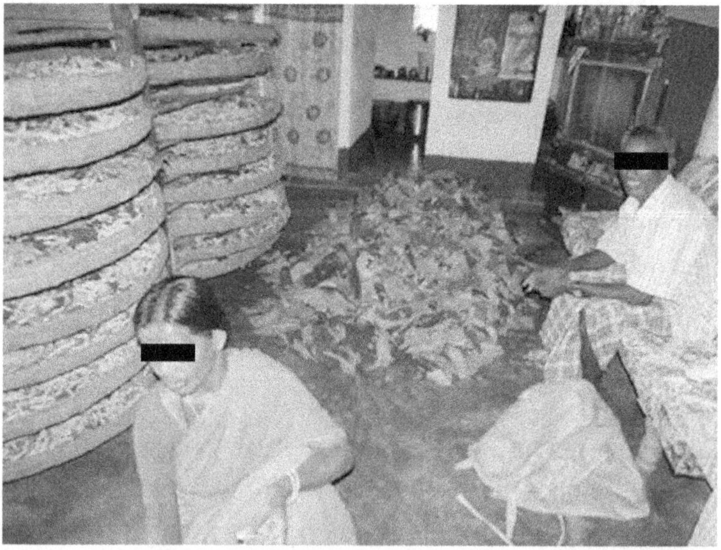

Figure 3: One of the homes where silkworms were being reared inside the house in vertical baskets in Chamarajanagar district, Karnataka, 2016

A traditional healer once explained to me that this is because silkworms can cause a rise in pitta among menstruating women. An aggravated pitta also impacts vāta, and if the same is continued month after month, it could disrupt the menstrual cycle, similar to what these women experienced.

Research on the impact of menstrual practices - The study titled "Rajaswala Paricharyā[14]: Effect on Menstrual Cycle and Its Associated Symptoms" by Dr. Pallavi Pai and team[15] reveals important insights on how the menstrual practices as per Āyurved can influence menstrual health.

The study was done on 30 healthy unmarried females in the age group of 18 to 24 years with a regular menstrual cycle. Subjects were asked to follow the rajaswala paricaryā paricryā for the first three days of their menstrual cycle for a period of six cycles. Menstrual history was taken before and after following the paricaryā. Observations were made on the follow-up of each regime every month, number of symptoms of each subject, and number of subjects showing the presence of each symptom.

Below is a table indicating the number of subjects showing the presence of symptoms before and after following the menstrual regime.

Table 5: Results of Rajaswala Paricharya study

Symptoms	Before	After	p-value
Pain in lower abdomen	28	3	$p<0.001$
Lower back ache	24	3	$p<0.001$
Pimples	20	5	$p<0.001$
Breast tenderness	1	0	$p<0.001$
Cramps in calf muscles	13	1	$p<0.001$
Loss of appetite	17	6	$p<0.01$
Hot flushes	12	5	$p=0.08$
Nausea/Vomiting	7	1	$p<0.001$
Constipation/Increased bowel movements	8	2	$p=0.07$
Increased frequency of micturition	6	1	$p<0.001$
Weakness	25	8	$p<0.001$
Headache/Migraine	11	1	$p<0.001$
Excitability/Irritability/ Depression	21	2	$p<0.001$

As indicated in the above table, the Chi-square test showed a significant decrease in the number of subjects showing the presence of symptoms.

In the area of menstrual research, such studies are a rarity, with most of the current research limiting itself to the use of menstrual products with the pre-determined intention of promoting sanitary napkins. Yet, no study to date has been able to prove beyond doubt that sanitary napkins have a positive impact on menstrual health or even hygiene for that matter. I have referred to more than 100 published research papers to arrive at this piece of information.[16]

Hopefully, with an increase in knowledge about Āyurved, there will be more such studies undertaken in the coming days which will be of actual benefit to women, rather than the pointless studies currently being done to promote menstrual products.

Experiencing the subtle

Cultural practices around menstruation came into being because of the understanding of the subtle forces that influence menstruation. But to experience this, it is necessary that we bring our menstrual cycle to a state of stability first. After all, we cannot see ripples on a water surface which is already disturbed. Women whose cycles are already disturbed and those who experience period pain or discomfort will most likely not be able to detect any change even if she breaks the above rules. The changes owing to not following the menstrual practices are difficult to detect immediately, given that it is very subtle, and unless we tune ourselves over a period of time, in all likelihood, these changes will go unnoticed.

From my own experience and that of several rural women who adhere to these menstrual practices, I assure you that it is possible to experience a period that is free from pain, discomfort, and aggravation of doṣas, just as mentioned in the ancient Āyurved texts. And once you are able to menstruate in such a way, you will begin to observe how the slightest thing, like someone's touch, can impact your period.

References for Chapter 2

1. Catamenial blood refers to menstrual blood
2. Shellac is the purified product of lac, the red, hardened secretion of the insect Laccifer lacca (lac beetle)
3. For details of the seven dhātus, refer the Notes section titled 'Dhātu'
4. The reference to menstrual practices in Suśruta Saṃhitā are taken from "An English Translation of The Suśruta Saṃhitā, edited by Kaviraj Kunja Lal Bhishagratna, Vol II, Nidana-Sthana
5. Collyrium, commonly called Kajal, is a medicated black eye liner, commonly used by women in Eastern countries to define the inner part of eyelids
6. Atreya. Ayurvedic Healing for Women, 1999
7. Caraka Saṃhita Sūtrasthāna, Ch. 20
8. Vāta prakṛti – body constitution which has a naturally dominant vāta doṣa
9. Hannoun AB1, Nassar AH, Usta IM, Zreik TG, Abu Musa AA. Effects of war on the menstrual cycle. Obstet Gynecol. 2007;109(4):929-932.
10. Ālocaka pitta is the sub-type of pitta doṣa which influences eyesight. See the section on 'Doṣa Sub-Types' in Notes for details.
11. Suśruta Samhita. Cikitsa Sthānam. Chapter XXIV – Anāgata-vadha-pratiśedaniya

12. It is likely that an assumption is made that the woman's period ends on day 3, making day 4 the ideal day for conceiving.

13. V Demidchik. Mechanisms of oxidative stress in plants: from classical chemistry to cell biology - Environmental and experimental botany, 2015

14. Rajaswala Paricaryā refers to the menstrual regime mentioned in Āyurved texts

15. Pallavi Pai, Sarita Bhutada, Prasad Pandkar. Rajaswala Paricharya: Effect on Menstrual Cycle and Its Associated Symptoms. IOSR Journal of Dental and Medical Sciences, Feb. 2015; 14(2): 82-87.

16. Joseph, Sinu. Menstruation: Rhetoric, Research, Reality. www.mythrispeaks.wordpress.com

17. Ranjaka pitta is a sub-type of Pitta doṣa, also called pigment Pitta from the circumstance of its imparting the characteristic colour to the lymph chyle as it is transformed into blood by coursing through the liver and spleen, where it is located

CHAPTER 3

MENSTRUAL BLOOD: IMPURE OR HIGHLY PURE?

"When I was a young girl and got my first period, it was part of my culture that a drop of the first blood would be consumed. The first blood was considered to bring good health and wellbeing."

These were the words of a woman aged around 80 years, who my team and I met at a cloth market in Manipur, in March 2015. She felt neither disgust nor shame in divulging this to strangers like us. She further informed us that in her culture (not practiced anymore), the cloth from the first menstrual bleeding was never discarded. It was stored away by the mother of the young girl and returned to her as a gift at the time of her marriage. This menstrual gift was thought to keep the girl and her family away from all evils and bring in good health.

The auspiciousness of menstrual blood is celebrated in Indian culture even today. In temples such as the Bhagavathi Devī temple in Chengannur (Kerala) and the Kāmākhya temple in Guwahati (Assam), where the Devī is believed to menstruate, the menstrual cloth is given to devotees as a prasād[1]. Devotees, especially male devotees, queue up for this cloth as it is thought to bring good luck, good health, protect from evil, and reign in prosperity.

Further, the symbolism of using the color red in rituals is associated with menstrual blood as the purest and most powerful aspect of the feminine. The red kuṅkuma[2] worn on the forehead by many Hindus is thus representative of the Śakti or primordial feminine force.

Menstrual blood banking

The healing aspect of menstrual blood is now coming to light even in modern medicine. The fairly new concept of menstrual blood banks is evidence that what was known in ancient Indian culture is slowly being recognized by modern scientists as well[3]. Menstrual blood, when banked before the age of 35 (pre-menopause), has the potential to be used in therapies requiring stem cells. Menstrual blood comprises the endometrium (lining of the uterus), which is formed and shed month after month. As a result, the stem cells from the menstrual blood are highly regenerative in nature. These stem cells can multiply rapidly and form new cells and tissues, making it a good source of stem cells in research for differentiation into different cells and use in regenerative medicine. The differentiation of menstrual stem cells into adipocytes, osteocytes, chondrocytes, hepatocytes, cardiomyocytes, and pancreatic cells has been studied[3]. Thus, the positive use of menstrual blood is acknowledged in modern science.

Menstruation for removal of toxins

During my interaction with adolescent girls across India, a common understanding was that menstruation causes the removal of accumulated toxins, thereby causing menstrual blood to be considered as impure blood. We must explore why women are often told that the reason for menstrual regulations has to do with becoming impure during menstruation. What are these toxins that are supposedly removed during menstruation?

The answer lies in Āyurved's concept of āmā, which is the term used by Āyurved to describe internal toxins. Āmā does not just refer to chemical or foreign substances that enter the body through the various pollutants that are knowingly and unknowingly consumed every day, but also to the residue of food that is partially digested or undigested and ends up rotting in the intestine. The result of improper digestion is the internal toxin referred to as āmā.

The Aṣṭāṅgahṛdaya text talks about āmā as the result of indulging in viruddha aśana (taking incompatible foods), adhyāsana (taking excess food), and ajīrṇa aśana (eating food which causes indigestion). This is said to develop the dreaded āmā doṣa, which is similar to poison. Hence, it is also called as āmā viśa (undigested food poison). The text suggests three techniques of apatarpaṇa (non-nourishment) to counter āmā. If āmā is not much, only laṅghana (fasting) will be sufficient; if it is moderate, laṅghana (fasting) and pācana (digestive drugs) are needed; if it is severe, then śodhana (pañcakarma therapy) is necessary, for these will expel out the doṣa and āmā from the very root.[4]

When āmā is excessive, it affects all the dhātus (tissue layers) and impairs the doṣas, resulting in disease. Excess āmā can also cause infertility when it affects the śukra dhātu, which is the seventh tissue layer corresponding to reproductive health. Āyurved's detox process called pañcakarma[5] is often prescribed for couples who have difficulty conceiving. Such processes help in eliminating āmā and restoring the body's natural balance. This is why Āyurved gives a lot of importance to the right diet to prevent the build-up of āmā.

In the parlance of modern medicine, it is likely that the role of āmā and its elimination can be understood through the study of the lymphatic system, which is considered as the body's secondary circulation system, which acts to drain waste from the body.[6] The lymphatic system is said to become active post ovulation and leading to menstruation (luteal phase), working to cleanse the body, thereby preventing menstrual problems. According to Dr. John Douillard[7], congested lymph brings with it the symptoms associated with the menstrual cycle, including breast swelling or tenderness, bloating, water retention, and/or breakouts. However, detailed research and studies on the lymphatic system in relation to menstruation are yet to be undertaken.

Pañcakarma techniques include five methods of detox—vamana (causing to eject the contents of the stomach by mouth), virecana (causing the evacuation of the intestines), nasya (causing elimination through nostrils and throat), anuvasana, and āsthāpana (medicated enemas meant to evacuate through the rectum). Interestingly, if āmā is excess, the process of menstruation causes the woman to clear out the toxins in ways similar to the results of the pañcakarma therapy. Thus, menstruation acts as a natural detox process offered to women by nature.

Āyurved considers menstruation as an important process because it causes the removal of accumulated āmā and cleanses the body. The association of menstruation with inner cleansing arises from this understanding. This process is exclusive to women because of the requirement of a healthy womb, in preparation for bearing a child. The primary paths for expelling internal toxins are through the intestines, urinary system, sinuses, lungs, and through the skin. The pushing out of āmā during menstruation manifests as problems at the time of menstruation in the form of acne, nausea, vomiting, loose bowel movements, sinus congestion (causing headaches), and gastric induced abdominal cramps that some women experience. The more the āmā, the greater the menstrual discomfort. Such discomforts are an indicator that needs to be taken seriously and corrected at an early stage through the right diet and an exercise routine that aids metabolism. It has been my experience with several women that the simple practice of avoiding food that is difficult to digest a week before and during menstruation, along with the daily practice of yōg and prāṇāyāma (except during menstruation), can positively change the way women experience menstruation. In addition to the right diet, regular practice of yōg and prāṇāyāma help to improve metabolism and digestion, thereby reducing āmā accumulation and consequently menstrual discomfort.

Thus, we see that the traditional knowledge of rural girls and women is not entirely incorrect—the process of menstruation does push out bodily toxins called āmā. But unlike popular perception, it is not the menstrual blood which is impure, but rather that the process of menstruation causes the release of impurities/āmā from the body.

This understanding is why rural women often explain the purpose of menstruation as something that cleanses the body and impacts the overall health of women, and not just limited to pregnancy or childbirth. Whereas, modern science has reduced menstruation to a process that is only necessary for bearing a child. The question 'If I don't intend to have children, do I need to bleed?' is, unfortunately, gaining popularity among so-called modern women. Consequently, period stopping pills and hysterectomy (removal of the uterus) are dangerously on the rise, compromising the overall health of women.

If women have this natural ability to remove āmā owing to menstruation, what about men? Boys and men do not have this advantage of voluntary removal of āmā through menstruation, and the result is that there is a greater prevalence of diseases among men, not to mention a shorter lifespan when compared to women. According to the United Nations World Population Prospects 2015 Revision, the worldwide average life expectancy of men is 69 years while it is 71 years for women. In India, it is 67 years for men and 70 years for women.

It is not uncommon to come across people who often feel sympathy for menstruating women owing to what they loosely term 'women's monthly problem'. But the fact is that it is this monthly event which gives women's health the decided advantage. For non-menstruating persons to have the equivalent cleansing of menstruation, they have to be regular in their exercise routine and be extra careful about their diet, because nature has not bestowed upon them the gift of a natural pañcakarma via menstruation.

When we hear people refer to menstrual blood as impure blood, we either dismiss the entire idea in order to make women feel empowered, or we become rigid in defense of an idea that has existed for so long. The answer lies somewhere in between. Such thought processes should not be dismissed without a thorough investigation of why it came into being, because hidden in it are important aspects of menstruation known to our ancestors, which will deepen our understanding of this subject.

References for Chapter 3

1. Prasād refers to a religious offering given to devotees
2. Kuṅkuma refers to a red pigment/vermillion used by Hindu women to make a round mark on the forehead and between parted hair
3. Khanjani S, Khanmohammadi M, Zarnani AH, Akhondi MM, Ahani A, Ghaempanah Z, Naderi MM, Eghtesad S, Kazemnejad S Comparative evaluation of differentiation potential of menstrual blood- versus bone marrow-derived stem cells into hepatocyte-like cells. PLoS One. 2014; 9(2):e86075.
4. Refer Aṣṭāṅgahṛdaya Sūtrasthāna
5. Pañcakarma is a treatment in Āyurved used to detox the body.
6. Brown P. Lymphatic system: unlocking the drains. Nature. 2005 Jul 28; 436(7050):456-8.
7. Dr. John Douillard. The Encyclopedia of Ayurvedic Massage, 2004.

Chapter 4

Menstrual Seclusion: What Women Need

> "My name is Nagarathnamma. I belong to the Katapanahatti Gollarahatti community. Some of us stay out of the house for up to three days during menstruation. So, we have to bathe and go to the toilet by the side of the road. There are no facilities to take a bath, and there is no room for us to stay outside. We have a lot of problems because of this."

These are the words of a woman belonging to the Golla community from Challakere town in Chitradurga district, Karnataka. In late 2014, there was a lot of media coverage and noise about how ancient practices of menstrual seclusion and patriarchy are causing problems for women in the Golla community. In all these media reports, reporters usually presented the voice of an agitated outsider and rarely had the women themselves speak. Media discussions were held on what should be done to these patriarchal men who force their women to follow such practices. The media interpretation seemed so obviously one-sided that my team and I decided to meet the Golla community and get first-hand information. What we learned was very different from what was projected.

When asked if they would agree to stay in their homes if the men asked them to stay, the Golla women spoke together and said,

> "No, no, we will not break this practice. It is an age-old tradition passed down from our ancestors, and we wish to follow it."

At the same time, the inconvenience caused was not lost on them. When asked what the solution to the problem is, another Golla woman, Shivamma, said:

> "We face a lot of difficulties when we stay outside our homes during menstruation. If it rains, we sit out with an umbrella. Please build a room for us with basic facilities, so that we can continue to follow our traditional practices." Echoing what she said, Nagarathnamma added, "We need better facilities while staying out. We need a room, a bathroom, a toilet, and water facility."

The Gollas

Gollas are a sheep-rearing community who live together in hamlets called hatti, across Tumkur, Hassan, and Chitradurga districts of Karnataka. While many Gollas today are well educated and well placed, there are still those who live in rural areas and follow their ancient practices very rigidly. We traveled to Gollarahattis[1] across Hassan and Chitradurga districts in Karnataka to understand their perspectives and practices around menstruation.

During the visit, we interacted with more than 300 women and men from six different hattis, explored the original reasons behind menstrual practices such as building menstrual huts, and filmed the voice of the Golla women. We learned that the reasons for practicing menstrual seclusion varied even among different Golla communities, with most of the reasons being quite practical.

Menstrual huts for privacy and health

Our first visit was to Thippaghatta Gollarahatti in Purehalli village, Arasikere Taluk, Hassan district. We spoke to some of the men and women in this community, with the help of the then panchayat[2] president. The men began by telling us that they feel awkward standing too close to other people because they smell like sheep. In this community, people often live in small houses as joint families, with 10-15 family members living under the same roof. The same space is extended and used for the sheep as well. When a woman menstruates, it becomes very inconvenient for her to remain in the same space as other male members of the family. They also said that menstruating women have lower immunity[3] and are likely to easily pick up diseases from the sheep if they shared the same space.

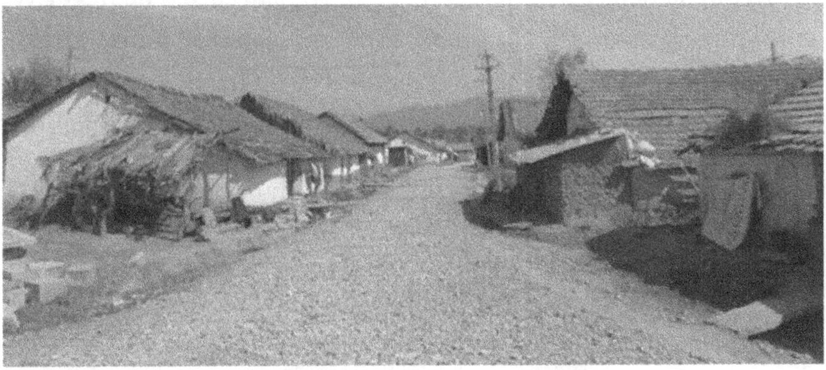

Figure 4: Homes of the Gollas in Arasikere, Hassan district, 2016

To avoid these difficulties, the community thoughtfully decided to create a separate space for menstruating women to bleed in privacy and without compromising their health. Not just any space, but a carefully planned menstrual hut that was built with medicinal plants and herbs familiar to that community. The leaves and plants used would not only keep the menstruating woman warm, but also protect her from snakes, poisonous insects, and prevent infection through their anti-bacterial and anti-fungal properties. The menstrual hut was also used by women who just gave birth to a child, in which case the mother and infant would remain in the hut for the first three months. The environment of the hut was thought to help them recover sooner and safeguard the newborn from getting infected by sheep-borne diseases. However, we were told that the women no longer retire to menstrual huts in this community but continue to follow seclusion by remaining in the backyard of their homes for the duration of their period.

In the local language, menstruating women and women who have just given birth are said to be in a state they call sūtakā. When the locals say that a woman is in sūtakā, it means that she is in a phase where she needs rest and special care. The negative connotations came with attempts to translate the word sūtakā to English, resulting in meanings indicating impurity or taboo. The understanding that menstruation and the months just after childbirth resulted in the loss of prāṇā (oxidative stress) is key to making sense of the seclusion practices and the special care with which specific medicinal plants are used for constructing menstrual huts. It is likely that these measures compensated for the loss of prāṇā and helped the woman recover sooner.

Menstrual huts to communicate with men

The following day, we interacted with Mr. Rudrappa, the leader of a hatti in Dodderi village, Chitradurga district, and he accompanied us to interact with women from Kasturi Thimmanahalli and Devera Urukunte villages. In his community too, menstrual huts were built not just for menstruating women but also for new mothers who just had a child. According to Mr. Rudrappa, the Golla men, being nomadic shepherds, would be gone for long periods of time to graze the sheep. At times, they would return only after a month or two. When the men returned, they would not know what condition their wife would be in, given that mobile phones were unheard of in the earlier times. For the man, seeing his wife in a menstrual hut meant that he should keep his distance and not indulge in sexual activities until she comes out of the hut. In these communities, it is understood that sexual intercourse during menstruation or just after a woman has given birth is harmful to the woman. This is also in line with what is mentioned in Āyurved texts.

It is important to note that the decision to have menstrual huts was made by the community, which included women. Such practices ensured rest for the women, as the men maintained a respectful distance until the sūtakā period was over.

What women want

Our next interaction was with the women introduced at the beginning of this chapter, who are from Kātapanahatti Gollarahatti, in Challakere town, Chitradurga district. Being a town, the houses where these women lived were cramped spaces, typical of low-income areas. The women we met were very religious and one of their husbands was a pūjāri[4]. Their homes were adjacent to a temple, and therefore, the practice of menstrual seclusion was still prevalent, as they strongly believed that menstruating women should not be near a temple (this practice is explained in Part II of this book). Here, the women were vocal about their difficulties owing to remaining outside the house during menstruation. And unlike the open spaces in villages, here, when a menstruating woman steps out of the house, she is literally on the road, where she has neither privacy nor facilities to manage her period. In spite of the difficulties, the women had no intention of discontinuing the practices. Instead, they requested us to build them special rooms with necessary facilities, where they could remain during menstruation.

It is interesting to note that at one point, the state government and local elected representatives did consider their request and built rooms called Krishna Kuteer for menstruating women. However, when the government changed, the practice was dismissed as superstition and the Krishna Kuteers were converted into Anganwadis[5] or other buildings. But this did not stop the menstruating women from using those spaces that were not converted, as we saw in Yerobahalli village. The Krishna Kuteer in Yerobahalli was constructed just outside the village because the village had a temple. Even though it is no longer fit for use, even now, menstruating women go to the kuteer and remain in the bushes just outside it. Needless to say, they put themselves at risk every month.

Even as I write this piece, in January 2020, the government of Karnataka introduced the anti-superstition law which aims to end the menstrual seclusion practices of the Golla women along with a few other practices. While the government and activists are determined to force the women to end this practice, the experiences and choice of the Golla women are not even considered, as indicated by this statement from one of the Golla women in an article on this subject:

"I was one of those who came out of the conservative practice. But soon I fell sick and the village pūjārappa suggested I should resume living separately outside the village during menstruation to recuperate. And this worked," says 24-year-old Thayamma.[6]

On one hand, there are women who have experienced the health effects of not following menstrual seclusion and wish to continue it, and on the other hand is a system that is determined to end the practice, not even bothering to respect the choice of those they intend to 'save'.

Is a ban the right answer?

In November 2018, a story emerged of the death of a 16-year-old girl in Tamil Nadu who was trapped in her menstrual hut during the cyclone Gaja. BBC did a story with the title "Cyclone Gaja: India girl segregated during period dies"[7]. Similar stories in Nepal led to much media noise, especially from the international community. The outside pressure on the Nepalese government was such that they had to criminalize the practice, called Chaupadi, in Nepal. After all, such stories make for great media sensation and keep menstrual activists busy.

While it is indeed unfortunate that young girls died in the menstrual hut, is it rocket science to realize that banning a practice is not going to bring it to an end? If anything, the entire practice is pushed underground, with menstruating women not having basic facilities while in seclusion, just as we witnessed in the case of the Golla women. A more sensible way of dealing with it would be to respect women's choice to follow their tradition and help them do it in a safer way. The root of the problem is not menstrual seclusion, although it makes for a great sad story of a third world country. The root of the problem is poverty.

If those practicing menstrual seclusion were not poor women from developing countries, their huts would be called Red Tents and would be applauded, as is currently happening. Red Tents are a movement in the west where women gather in red-colored tents set up in public spaces to take time out, share their stories, rest, and listen to each other. These meetings are organized around the lunar calendar and take place on the new moon or full moon. While those who visit the Red Tent might themselves not be aware, the reason for meeting around the new moon or full moon is because it is traditionally linked to menstrual bleeding in sync with the moon's cycle. There is also an online Red Tent Directory (www.redtentdirectory.com) for women in Europe to find their nearest red tent. As of 2016[8], the site listed 57 active groups across England, Wales, and Northern Ireland. Red Tents apparently help women honor the menstrual/feminine cycle. Don't be surprised if you see women with red bindis on their foreheads, bangles on their hands, swaying to tribal music, and using pictures of Hindu deities for decoration!

For the modern western world that is starved of a cultural acceptance of menstruation, movements like Red Tent are an exotic experience. For the Indian and Nepalese women who actually need it and to whom it belongs, it is a basic right that is snatched away in the name of women's empowerment.

References for Chapter 4

1. The hamlets where the Golla community live is called Gollarahatti
2. In India, villages are grouped into Panchayats for administrative purposes.
3. Indigenous sciences recognize that menstruating women pick up diseases more easily owing to a reduced immunity during this time. Therefore, care is taken to prevent her from coming in contact with other people.
4. Pūjāri is one who performs pūja in a temple
5. An Anganwadi is a nursery for children below the age of 5 years.
6. Pailoor, Anitha. It's period: Karnataka's anti-superstition law ends Kadugolla custom. Deccan Herald, January 24, 2020
7. BBC News. 'Cyclone Gaja: India girl segregated during period dies'. 21 Nov 2018
8. Telegraph: Why Women Are Gathering In 'Red Tents' across the UK, by Cathy Wallace (2 Feb 2016)

CHAPTER 5

SPORTS AND MENSTRUATION: WHY IT DOESN'T HAVE TO BE PAINFUL

A modern-day sportswoman remains in the prime of her sports career until the age of about 30-35 years. After that, her body begins to give up. In comparison, a female Kalaripayattu (traditional martial art from Kerala) performer continues well into her later years. The example of the Padma Śrī awardee Meenakshi Amma, aged 76 and still wielding a sword, is testimony to it [1]. Similarly, women trained in traditional dance forms like Bharatanatyam are known to perform on stage well into their eighties.

The big difference in the traditional and modern sports/ dance practice is simply this—all traditional martial arts and dance forms originating in India insisted that the female players/ performers take time off during menstruation. Whereas, in modern sports, women are told to battle it out and be equal to men. And the result is frequent injury, troubled menstruation, difficulty during childbirth, and under-performance in the chosen sport.

Menstruation does not have to be a hurdle for women who are into sports or other physically demanding careers; instead, it can become their biggest advantage, provided the management and coaches stop behaving as though the bodies of female sportspersons are the same as that of male sportspersons, and instead encourage sportswomen to work in sync with their menstrual cycle.

In 2016, I set out to understand how sports impacted menstruation and if menstruation could impact sports performance. To gain a deeper understanding, I interviewed women from diverse sports backgrounds, such as athletics, long jump, powerlifting, gymnastics, sports bike racing, kabbadi, and traditional martial arts, such as Capoeira, Kalaripayattu, Silambam. To understand the Āyurvedic perspective, Dr. Ramya Bhat, an Āyurved physician based in Bengaluru, was consulted. This chapter summarizes what I learned and what modern-day sportswomen can do to ensure that their health is not negatively impacted by their choice in career.[2]

How doṣas impact performance

If you have read the chapter 'Understanding Menstrual Practices through Āyurved', you will know by now that every woman's menstrual cycle and personality is specific to her doṣa type. This is true even for sportswomen.

Sportswomen with vāta prakṛti - Women whose body constitution is dominated by vāta doṣa tend to have more menstrual problems and injuries, especially if they engage in physical activity during or just prior to menstruation and do not take necessary precautions to prevent vāta aggravation. As a result, sportswomen with vāta prakṛti are more likely to have amenorrhea (delayed menses), dysmenorrhea (pain during menses), and are prone to frequent injuries. By the sheer will of their mind, they might even overcome the cramps, pain, and disorientation. But the long-term effect of the continuous aggravated vāta could result in difficulty in conceiving, difficulty during childbirth, and early osteoporosis.

Sportswomen with pitta prakṛti - Any aggravation in vāta doṣa can also result in a disturbance in pitta doṣa. Pitta dominant women tend to feel too much body heat and sweating just before their period and excessive physical exercise can worsen it. Usually, heavy menstrual bleeding is characteristic of a pitta prakopa; so is anemia. When it comes to sports, pitta women are highly competitive, focused, and determined, but they burn out and feel exhausted sooner than others if necessary precautions are not taken to prevent pitta aggravation.

Sportswomen with kapha prakṛti - Kapha prakṛti women actually benefit from sports as exercise increases the vāta and pitta, thereby balancing out the heavy feeling of kapha. Such women might even feel that they perform better when they have their period, as told to me by one athlete. Kapha prakṛti women have greater endurance and can experiment with pushing their limits. They make great marathoners, sprinters, and wrestlers.

Most women are a combination of two or more doṣas with one dominant doṣa. A combination of kapha-pitta might be very well suited for sports and intensive physical exercises, as it combines kapha's endurance and strength with pitta's focus and competitiveness. Determining the dominant doṣa and prakṛti of sportswomen, especially at an early age, can be of immense help when it comes to planning the type of practice, food, and even type of sport that would be most suited to them.

Menstrual difficulties among sportswomen

Paula Radcliffe[3], a British long-distance runner, once said: "Sports has not learned how to deal with elite athletes' periods."

In the present day and age, with all the advancement in science, the impact of menstruation on sportswomen is woefully under-studied. Often, sportswomen are told to suppress menstruation using period postponing pills, consume painkillers for cramps, and even take hormones to make their bodies more masculine in order to perform better. This, coupled with the utter lack of knowledge of what causes sportswomen to experience such pain and menstrual difficulties, makes this topic extremely important for sportswomen. In the following paragraphs, the menstrual problems faced by sportswomen, the cause of menstrual difficulties as per Āyurved, and the solutions from indigenous knowledge systems that will enable women to work with their cycles to have better health without compromising on performance will be outlined.

As per Āyurved, vāta doṣa is responsible for sending signals to initiate movement of hormones that cause ovulation and menstruation. However, if vāta is vitiated, this sending and receiving of signals to trigger hormones could be affected, resulting in various menstrual disorders. Let's take a look at the different menstrual disorders and how it might be caused among sportswomen.

1. Amenorrhea (missed period for 6 months or more)

Mary Cain, who qualified for the 2013 world championships as a 17-year-old and was considered a once-in-a-generation star, is an unfortunate example of what female sportspersons have to endure. Mary Cain's male coaches (who were part of Nike's training program) were convinced that she had to get "thinner, and thinner, and thinner", until her body started breaking down. Her period stopped for three years, she broke five different bones owing to osteoporosis, and cut herself in an attempt to commit suicide. In her own words,

> "I wasn't even trying to make it to Olympics anymore, I was just trying to survive."

It must have taken her immense courage and suffering to publicly say,

> "They are not acknowledging that there is a systemic crisis in which young girls' bodies are being ruined by an emotionally and physically abusive system." [4]

While Mary Cain eventually spoke out against this systemic abuse, many female athletes might still be silent on how sports have altered their bodies. Amenorrhea is a common problem among sportswomen and a result of over-exercising. Recent studies[5] mention that female athletes may experience difficulties in achieving pregnancy due to athletic amenorrhea (AA). For professional female athletes, the incidence of athletic amenorrhea (AA) is particularly high, at a rate of 65-69% in athletes, dancers, and distance runners compared with 2-5% in normal women.[6] The underlying mechanisms of AA remain unknown in modern medicine. However, with the help of Āyurved, it is possible to understand the cause of AA.

During week 1 & 2 of the menstrual cycle, which is the week after menstruation and leading to ovulation, there is a rise in the levels of the hormone estrogen. During this time, an aggravated vāta due to over-exercising can affect the menstrual cycle in the following ways:

- ✦ If vāta is already disrupted at the beginning of the first week, then estrogen levels do not rise as expected, resulting in anovulation (no ovulation).
- ✦ If vāta is disturbed during the second week, it prevents signals from being sent to reduce estrogen (estrogen levels peak at ovulation and should reduce after that). Therefore, estrogen levels keep rising and there will be no menstruation. This results in amenorrhea. In Āyurved, amenorrhea is understood to be a deficiency disease due to vāta. Lack of body fat and too much exercise can bring it about, which is why athletic women often fail to get their period.

2. Dysmenorrhea (menstrual cramps/pain/discomfort)

When Chinese swimmer Fu Yuanhui won a bronze medal for the women's 100m backstroke at the 2016 Olympic Games, she made headlines for telling the world that she was on her period on that day[7]. An interviewer found her doubled over and grimacing. She asked Fu if she was in pain, to which Fu replied,

> "Actually, my period started last night, so I'm feeling pretty weak and really tired."

And this, the world applauded because, apparently, she broke a taboo by talking about menstruation publicly. Did it occur to no one that her pain probably had to do with swimming during menstruation? Instead of being applauded, she needed help from a system that understood the impact of swimming while menstruating. The other example is of Jazmin Sawyers, the British long jumper, who pulled out of a competition because of chronic period pain.[8]

During my interview with a former athlete from India who was a South Asian Games champion in long jump, she said:

"Couple of times during the Asian championships, I was expecting to win a gold, but due to my periods, I could not jump as well as I had expected and could only win bronze... My body gets heavy, exhausted sooner than normal days. During training, it wasn't much of an issue, but during competitions, it is totally demotivating."

The knowledge of dysmenorrhea among female sportspersons and how it can be prevented is as good as non-existent in modern medicine. As Jazmin Sawyers said,[9]

"I have a concoction of painkillers and anti-inflammatories that, to be honest, usually work, and sometimes don't. We still don't know why the pain is so bad, and we're still trying to optimize a management plan for it."

From the perspective of Āyurved, the cause of dysmenorrhea can be understood. Vāta doṣa has five subtypes[10] which govern movements in different parts of the body. The subtype which is responsible for downward movement of urination, excretion, menstrual blood, and childbirth is called apāna vāyu. It is located in the lower part of the body, near the genitals. During menstruation, apāna vāyu moves downward to facilitate the flowing out of menstrual blood. Dysmenorrhea can result from any of the below causes:

- ✦ Improper diet just before or during menses - Among most women suffering from menstrual pain and cramps, dysmenorrhea occurs due to consumption of unwholesome food just before or during menses and incomplete digestion, which causes gastric problems. When apāna is acting downward during menstruation, it pushes out the toxins and excessive gas accumulated in the body. If the toxins are more due to unhealthy food habits, menstruating women experience greater pain and cramps.

- Excessive physical exercise just before or during menstruation - Among sportswomen, vāta aggravation happens mainly due to excessive physical exercise just before or during menstruation. Since vāta is associated with movement, excessive movement disturbs the natural balance of vāta. Menstruation is a process where vāta is naturally predominant. Therefore, putting the body through excessive physical exercise during menstruation aggravates the vāta, causing menstrual discomfort.
- Blockage or upward movement of apāna - During menstruation, if women undertake activities which alter the downward direction of apāna or temporarily stop its downward movement, then they are quite likely to experience menstrual cramps due to apāna being blocked or pulled in an opposite direction. For example, swimming or being underwater for long will temporarily stop the menstrual flow (we can observe this temporary stopping of menses even when we take a long shower); inverted postures during Yōg āsana or gymnastics could reverse apāna; activities such as long jump during menstruation, which temporarily lifts the body against gravity, might also cause apāna to act against gravity, causing menstrual pain.

3. Menorrhagia (heavy menstrual bleeding) and anemia

In 2015, universities in the UK undertook a research study titled "The Prevalence and Impact of Heavy Menstrual Bleeding (Menorrhagia) among Elite and Non-Elite Athletes".[11] They studied 789 participants via an online survey and 1073 via face-to-face interviews at the 2015 London Marathon. The results revealed that 54% of those surveyed online reported heavy menstrual bleeding and 37% of Elite athletes also reported heavy menstrual bleeding. Overall, 32% of exercising females reported a history of anemia. Only a minority (22%) had sought medical advice.

According to Āyurved, menorrhagia and anemia are conditions that occur due to vitiated pitta doṣa. Pitta can get vitiated due to overeating of meat, hot, spicy, sour, or salty food, resulting in improper digestion. Women who consume non-vegetarian food regularly have a higher chance of heavy menstrual bleeding, since meat increases pitta. Any vitiation in vāta can also cause pitta to increase. Thus, excessive exercising combined with a meat-based diet, especially on the days just before and during menstruation, could result in heavy menstrual bleeding. It is more likely among women who have a pitta prakṛti.

Aggravated pitta could also result in nutritional deficiency anemia, i.e. a hemoglobin count of less than 12mg/dL. In such cases, the aggravated pitta results in improper absorption of nutrients, resulting in the lack of iron content in the blood. Anemia can cause weakness, exhaustion, and lack of concentration. In Āyurved, treatment of anemia involves pacifying and balancing the pitta, so that the body is able to absorb the nutrients in food, even if iron supplements are not consumed.

4. Polycystic Ovarian Syndrome (PCOS)

In an article titled "Role of Testosterone for the Female Athlete", coach and author Amber Larsen looks at research done to study the effect of exercise on female testosterone. She writes[23]:

"A main effect occurred for exercise with the post-testosterone concentration being greater than pre-exercise, although pre-exercise versus 30 minutes after was not different. All testosterone hormonal concentrations immediately post-exercise greatly exceeded the baseline levels[...] So basically, when you work out, your body is either making more testosterone or destroying less of it. Either way, you end up with a higher total level right after you exercise."

According to Dr. Ramya Bhat, an increase in testosterone could happen when women are involved in male-dominated sports, such as wrestling or weightlifting, that require more muscle strength. Testosterone is known to play an important role in muscle strength and sexual libido for women. Usually, testosterone levels peak only during ovulation, and even then, it is much lesser compared to the testosterone levels in men. But when triggered at other times, the increased testosterone could result in Polycystic Ovarian Syndrome (PCOS), which is characterized by excessive facial hair, masculine voice, and infertility or, in other words, hyperandrogenism.

Studies indicate that PCOS is overrepresented among Olympic sportswomen,[12] causing them reproductive dysfunction. But instead of considering this as a problem and finding ways to prevent sportswomen from having to experience reproductive problems, the sporting world is busy trying to explain why increased testosterone levels improve sporting performance among female athletes![13] Strangely enough, there are studies that suggest that even mild forms of hyperandrogenism like PCOS may be beneficial for physical performance and could play a role in the recruitment of women to competitive sports activities.[14]

Women's bodies have not only been misunderstood, but have also been exploited in a way that is unfair, disrespectful, and without any consideration for her reproductive preference.

5. Injuries while menstruating

A BBC article by Aimee Lewis[15] quotes several sportswomen sharing their experience of how injuries during menstruation have affected their performance. The article says:

In 2009, Anne Keothavong became the first British woman in 16 years to be ranked inside the world's top 50 but hers was a career troubled by knee injuries sustained when she was menstruating.

> "It does affect you, there's no doubt about it. I had ACL injuries on both knees and both times when I fell over it was that time of the month," says the 31-year-old.

Studies indicate that sports injuries are more common in women than in men.[16] Women have more body fat, greater flexibility, wider pelvis, lighter bone, and less muscle strength, and are more prone to miserable malalignment syndrome than men.[17] In particular, female athletes are known to be exposed to more sports injuries due to insufficient energy utilization, bone loss, and menstrual disturbances.[18] Āyurved can explain why this is so.

Women are more easily susceptible to injuries if they engage in excessive physical exercise during menstruation. This is because exercise aggravates the already dominant vāta in a menstruating woman. In healthy women, vāta doṣa maintains the equilibrium of tissues, bone density, and strength of joints. During instances when vāta is naturally predominant, like in the case of menstruation, the chance of injuries becomes higher. Dr. Ramya Bhat says that girls who are introduced early into sports, such as at the age of 6 or 7 and are not guided on measures to prevent vāta aggravation, become highly susceptible to weak joints and injuries by the time they are 18 or 20 years old.

This is the reason why a menstrual leave was strictly prescribed for female classical dancers or martial art performers in India. Traditionally, in most cultures, menstruating women were told not to engage in excessive physical exercise. Somehow, being modern has meant that we dismiss everything ancient without a thorough investigation of the reasons. So, it has been the trend that in the race to be equal to men, women have been trained to act like their bodies are no different from that of men.

6. Disorientation during menstruation

Balance ability has been reported to be one of the factors associated with sports injuries.[19] Balance is affected by various systems such as the sensory, motor, and central nervous systems. Sex hormone receptors are found in the bone, skeletal muscle, ligaments, and the nervous system.[20] Understanding the relationship between balance ability and hormonal changes in females is important in terms of injury prevention. Studies indicate that the menstrual cycle affects the static balance of healthy women and that during the menstrual cycle, the intensity of balance exercises in females should be carefully controlled for injury prevention.[21]

This aspect of menstruation impacting the sensory organs is well understood in Āyurved. Vāta controls the sensory perceptions and coordination of the sense organs. During menstruation, even simple activities like driving a car would seem a little daunting, as the ability to assess distances become clouded, due to the dominance of vāta doṣa. Expecting a sportswoman to perform during menses is like expecting us to do the same when we experience a jet lag.

When I interviewed Aishwarya Mannivannan, a national & international Silambam[22] Champion, and asked if she faced any difficulty in hand-eye coordination during menstruation, this is what she had to say in response:

> "I have not faced any specific issues so far. During menstruation, I feel that the fatigue and body pain sometimes lead to lack of concentration. In Silambam, even a momentary lapse in focus can lead to injury and one hitting themselves. So, during my period, I have faced situations occasionally, where I have lost concentration due to tiredness and failed to keep up my regular rhythm in movement."

Like Ms. Mannivannan, other sportswomen who were interviewed too did not make much of poor concentration or lack of coordination during menstruation, although they might have experienced it. Their sheer mental effort and determination to overcome this temporary disorientation are indeed laudable.

Most women do not distinguish between overall fatigue during menstruation and specific problems like sensory disorientation. Further, in the absence of sufficient evidence that supports it in modern science, it is not surprising that disorientation during menstruation is largely unnoticed. But, think of how much it could impact a sport in which hand-eye coordination or assessing distances can make all the difference in winning and losing.

7. Side effects of period postponing pills

Let's look at the incident of what happened to English middle-distance runner Jessica Judd, who failed to make it to the 800m semi-finals in the 2013 Moscow World Championships. This happened because the British Athletics medics prescribed Norethisterone (period postponing pill) to delay the onset of her period. In her own words:

"I can run so much quicker. I think I'm in 1.58 shape, so to run over two minutes is just a disaster in my opinion[...] It was a horrible situation which taught me a lot."[3]

Commenting on this, Paula Radcliff, who set the marathon world record in 2002, told BBC Sport:

> "It wasn't the first time they'd given it to an athlete and it hadn't helped. I would argue it's a lack of learning. Too often in sport, doctors are men and they don't understand.
>
> I knew from experience that this norethisterone drug made things a hundred times worse. Jo Pavey knew that, others knew that, but it seemed that nobody within British Athletics had written that down, in terms of 'we won't give that to other young athletes'. They were still trying it, that's what frustrated me.
>
> They tried it because that's what medical science was saying you should do in that situation, but they knew that it hadn't worked because athletes had told them 'I feel worse'. Yet Jess was still given it."

The article further reports that Radcliffe called for more studies to be done on the impact of the menstrual cycle on female performance—drawing on the experience of elite athletes, such as herself and Jo Pavey, who have "tried to do things to control their period" throughout their careers.

Period postponing pills are commonly prescribed for sportswomen whose event might coincide with the period. These pills contain the synthetic version of the hormone progesterone. Remember that for a period to occur, progesterone levels naturally drop. So, by keeping up the levels of progesterone artificially, menstruation is delayed for as long as the pill is consumed. Since progesterone is associated with the effects of PMS such as bloating and stomach cramps, these become the short-term side effects of consuming period postponing pills.

8. Long-term impact

Frequent use of period postponing pills and excessive exercise during menstruation can have long-term health impacts, even if it doesn't show in obvious ways immediately. A continuous aggravation of vāta can result in early osteoporosis, as the bone density is reduced when vāta is vitiated. A woman whose vāta doṣa has been vitiated and has become pregnant is likely to face difficulties during childbirth and labor. Since apāna vāyu's downward movement is the force that pushes the fetus out, any disturbance in it or change in its direction can make labor very difficult.

Preventing menstrual difficulties among sportswomen

When women go out there and play for their nation, they put their health at risk. The solution obviously does not lie in asking a woman not to participate in sports, but rather in acknowledging that menstruation does have an impact and taking measures to prevent health risks for sportswomen. Āyurved's knowledge of menstruation can play an important role in helping sportswomen perform better.

There are ways to tap into the body's natural intelligence, to work with the menstrual cycle and not against it, to overcome menstrual difficulties. Indigenous knowledge systems that have worked with women dancers and martial art performers have a lot to offer the modern-day sportswomen. Given below are four such examples from India's ancient knowledge systems.

1. Preventing vāta prakopa

The most likely doṣa imbalance for sportswomen is vāta prakopa (vāta aggravation), due to over-exercising. Āyurved and traditional martial arts like Kalaripayattu recommend that women refrain from exercising 3-4 days during their period. An ideal world would be one where women's bodies and their rhythms are taken into consideration before planning events for them. However, given that most sporting events will not take a woman's period into account, women will have to play during their period in case of a major tournament. But, until that happens, it is best to avoid practicing or playing during one's period. Exercising during menstruation can cause injuries more easily. So, if your period comes just before a big tournament, the smart thing to do is to stay away from training, lest your injuries keep you from performing during the event.

Dr. Ramya Bhat has the following advice for women to prevent aggravation of vāta while exercising (this is especially important for women who have a vāta prakṛti):

- Avoid food that further aggravates vāta. Food that is cold, raw, or dry tends to increase vāta. Warm and well-cooked food is advised.
- During the week just before menstruation, more attention needs to be paid to what you eat, as vāta and pitta rise during this time. Having vāta suppressing food is recommended during this time.
- Āyurved suggests oil massage as a good remedy to prevent vāta aggravation and resulting injuries. However, this is not to be done during menstruation.
- In traditional sports like Kushti (Indian wrestling) and Kalaripayattu (Indian martial art), the players oil and massage their body before practice. Oiling makes the body more supple and flexible, lubricates the joints, reducing injury, and keeps vāta from aggravating. In Kalari, the full body is massaged with gingelly oil or special medicated oils to treat specific sprains, and the head is drenched with coconut oil to pacify excessive pitta (heat). Note that oil massages are not recommended during menstruation, as it might interfere with the natural dominance of vāta and pitta during menstruation.

To determine the type of food and suitable oils for specific body types, it is best to consult an experienced Āyurved physician.

2. Exercising: how much is too much?

Āyurved prescribes that physical exercise should only be done to half of an individual's capacity. When an individual starts breathing from his/her mouth, it is an indication that he/she needs to stop. Interestingly, all sportswomen I interviewed flout this rule on a regular basis. Modern-day sports training pushes athletes to exceed their limit, assuming that this is how endurance is built. A better method of training to build endurance is explained by Kutti Krishnan Gurukkal, a Kalaripayattu master from Kerala, who has been training students for over 25 years in this ancient martial art. This is what he told me during a telephone interview:

> "The exercises in Kalaripayattu should be done only for 50% of that person's capacity. Whereas in modern sports, if he can run one km, we make him run till he gets exhausted. In Kalaripayattu, we first train the legs, then we move to the upper body, and so on. Then, finally, you bring the entire body to a stage where he/she can perform without getting exhausted. But we do not begin by forcing the child to keep running till they exhaust themselves. If the body has to be prepared to fight for 3-4 hours a day, it can't be done in a short time by pushing people to exhaust themselves."

3. Food: meat-based or plant-based?

Modern sportspersons, some even vegetarians, switch to a meat-based diet, given the belief that it provides the needed nutrition, especially proteins. But, is this really what an exhausted body needs? Indiscriminate consumption of nutrition without considering the state of the body can do more harm than good. This aspect is considered in indigenous martial arts. In the words of Kutti Krishnan Gurukkal:

> "In modern sports, when a sportsperson is exhausted and worn out, we bring him in a stretcher and immediately feed him with broiler chicken! What your body needs at that time is glucose. By feeding them meat, we give extra work

to the body and digestive system. That's why traditionally in Kalari, we give them paal kanji (sweetened milk & rice porridge); this supplies the needed glucose. But if we give them meat, it is hard for them to digest, and they become easily prone to disease."

In Kalaripayattu, the prescribed diet is vegetarian; fish is allowed, but meat is prohibited, and everything is cooked in ghee (clarified butter) to ease digestion. For women especially, a plant-based diet is all the more important a week before and during menstruation, since meat can really worsen the situation by increasing pitta and put undue pressure on the digestive system. Besides, as Dr. Ramya Bhat says, "Women sportspersons need to ensure that they have enough iron and calcium intake. This is more important for them than protein because menstruation could result in iron and calcium deficiency."

4. Sports medicine: how about equipping the sportsperson instead of relying on a whole troupe of specialists?

The way of modern medicine is to compartmentalize everything. As a result, there is a specialist for every part of the body, happy to draw strict boundaries of their individual expertise. Therefore, sports medicine today comprises a team of specialty physicians and surgeons, athletic trainers, physical therapists, nutritionists, psychologists, coaches, other personnel, and, of course, the athlete. Specialties within sports medicine could further include cardiology, pulmonology, orthopedic surgery, psychiatry, exercise physiology, biomechanics, and traumatology.

Refreshingly different is the way of kalari cikitsā. At the last leg of kalaripayattu training, the student is trained in kalari cikitsā or marma cikitsā (cikitsā means treatment). Students are taught about their body, how to treat cuts/injuries, and how to do a specialized massage to recover from aches and sprains. A kalaripayattu expert depends on none but himself/herself to be at the best health and to heal from injuries.

Understanding the opponent's body and mind as well as training your own body and mind is an essential part of kalaripayattu. While modern sports promote aggression, kalaripayattu and kushti, even though more deadly in nature, train the student to be in control of the mind. Controlled aggression can indeed be more useful than mindless and restless aggression.

Thus, every specialty possible is taught holistically in kalaripayattu, equipping the student to deal with every situation, be it physical or mental. Imagine what would happen if we trained modern sportspersons, especially women, the same way?

Menstruation - the advantage for sportswomen

David Bock, a teacher of Wadokai Aikido and an acupuncturist, writes in his article 'Female Martial Artists & Amenorrhea'[24]:

> "Female martial artists, as with all serious female athletes, have a distinct advantage over their male counterparts in one very crucial area: The menstrual cycle.
>
> This monthly occurrence provides a window into the functioning of the female body. The smooth functioning of the cycle and periods indicates smooth functioning in many internal dynamics of the body. Sharp cramps, excessive bleeding, and inconsistent or missed periods can

> be an indication that the body is not functioning at its peak performance[...]
>
> Men do not have this obvious signal, and are more prone to overtraining to the point of permanent damage."

For female sportspersons, menstruation can be an advantage, both for their overall health and for their performance. Modern women have been taught to view menstruation as a monthly inconvenience to be overlooked and set aside as they climb the ladder of professional and personal success. As one sportswoman I interviewed put it, "According to me, this period thing is overrated."

Unlike men, who only get to know once the damage has been done, women are given obvious signals early on via menstruation. The knowledge required to identify these early signs of ill health will give sportswomen an undue advantage in preventing bodily damage and improving performance—provided they learn how to decode their period.

Menstruation does not have to become a painful hurdle for sportswomen, and they can be taught to train in sync with the rhythms of their menstrual cycle. But implementing this requires a massive change in mindset at all levels—from sports management to coaches to sports medics to the sportswoman herself. As the saying goes, "It takes effort to win the game, but it takes courage to change the game."

References for Chapter 5

1. Six decades on, 74-year-old Padma Shri awardee Gurukkal still swirling the sword. Hindustan Times. 29 January 2018.
2. This chapter originally appeared as an article in www.indiafacts.com, written by the author, titled 'Sports and Menstruation: Exploring Indigenous Knowledge', Part I and II. It has been reproduced here with modifications and additions.
3. Paula Radcliffe: Sport has not learned about periods. BBC Sport, 22 Jan 2015
4. Mary Cain. I was the fastest girl in America, Until I joined Nike. Nov 7, 2019.
5. Xiong RH, Wen SL, Wang Q, Zhou HY, Feng S. Morphological and molecular variations induce mitochondrial dysfunction as a possible underlying mechanism of athletic amenorrhea. Exp Ther Med. 2018 Jan;15(1):993-998. Epub 2017 Nov 8.
6. Warren MP and Perlroth NE: The effects of intense exercise on the female reproductive system. J Endocrinol 170: 3-11, 2001.
7. Uninhibited Chinese Swimmer, Discussing her Period, Shatters another barrier. New York Times, Aug 2016.
8. Jazmin Sawyers: period pain forced me to pull out of Boston long jump. The guardian. Jun 2017.
9. Jazmin Sawyers. "This is important. Period". www.worldathletics.org, 25 Jan 2018
10. See the Notes section titled "Subtypes of Doṣa" to know more about the vāta sub-types

11. Bruinvels G, Burden R, Brown N, Richards T, Pedlar C (2016). The Prevalence and Impact of Heavy Menstrual Bleeding (Menorrhagia) in Elite and Non-Elite Athletes. PLoS ONE 11(2): e0149881.

12. Hagmar M, Berglund B, Brismar K, Hirschberg AL. Hyperandrogenism may explain reproductive dysfunction in female Olympic athletes. Med Sci Sports Exerc. 2009;41:1241–1248.

13. Wood RI, Stanton SJ. Testosterone and sport: current perspectives. Horm Behav. 2012;61:147–155.

14. Stéphane Bermon, Eric Vilain, Patrick Fénichel, Martin Ritzén, Women With Hyperandrogenism in Elite Sports: Scientific and Ethical Rationales for Regulating, The Journal of Clinical Endocrinology & Metabolism, Volume 100, Issue 3, 1 March 2015, Pages 828–830

15. Lewis, Aimee. Curse or Myth – do periods affect performance? BBC, 22-Jan-2015

16. Ristolainen L, Heinonen A, Waller B, et al.: Gender differences in sport injury risk and types of injuries: a retrospective twelve-month study on cross-country skiers, swimmers, long-distance runners and soccer players. J Sports Sci Med, 2009, 8: 443–451.

17. Casey E, Hameed F, Dhaher YY: The muscle stretch reflex throughout the menstrual cycle. Med Sci Sports Exerc, 2014, 46: 600–609.

18. Barrack MT, Gibbs JC, De Souza MJ, et al.: Higher incidence of bone stress injuries with increasing female athlete triad-related risk factors: a prospective multisite study of

exercising girls and women. Am J Sports Med, 2014, 42: 949–958

19. Nadler SF, Malanga GA, DePrince M, et al.: The relationship between lower extremity injury, low back pain, and hip muscle strength in male and female collegiate athletes. Clin J Sport Med, 2000, 10
20. Griffin LY, Agel J, Albohm MJ, et al.: Noncontact anterior cruciate ligament injuries: risk factors and prevention strategies. J Am Acad Orthop Surg, 2000, 8: 141–150.
21. BJ Lee, KH Cho, WH Lee. The effects of the menstrual cycle on the static balance in healthy young women. Journal of physical therapy science. 2017
22. Silambam is a weapon-based traditional martial art from Tamil Nadu, India
23. Larsen, Amber. The role of testosterone for the female athlete. www.breakingmuscle.com
24. Bock, David. Female Martial Artists and Amenorrhea. www.fightingarts.com

CHAPTER 6

CELESTIAL INFLUENCE ON MENSTRUAL CYCLES

What influences and causes menstruation to occur?

Is there a pattern to the way it occurs?

Is it predictable?

These questions have plagued me for years. Most people who study menstrual cycles rarely look beyond the vague answers offered by modern medical science. According to gynecologists, an adult woman's monthly period could occur anywhere between 21 to 35 days and between 21 to 45 days for adolescent girls. The wide unexplained variation does not seem to bother many. Perhaps because it allows irregular cycles to be considered as normal. But for someone looking at it from the perspective of Āyurved and other indigenous sciences, regularity and predictability in the menstrual cycle is everything. If the monthly period does not come as expected, it is an early indicator of menstrual or other health problems that could occur if nothing is done to prevent it. This is why it is of utmost importance that women learn to observe patterns in their cycle.

Of all the chapters I have written until this point, this one was the most complex. The difficulty is because it requires us to not only bring attention to minute micro details that influence each woman's body differently but also requires us to understand the macro details that cast an influence on the day-to-day functioning of human beings. In other words, it requires us to understand the celestial influence on the female menstrual cycle, which includes the influence of the Sun, the Moon, other planets, constellations, and their transitions.

When it comes to information about celestial influence on menstrual cycles, there are those who say that women should bleed in sync with the amāvāsyā (new moon) to be healthy. Similarly, there are some who say that it is the pūrṇimā (full moon) which is the right time to bleed. I myself had thought one or the other to be true at different points in my study. However, when I started charting my cycle over the last 16 months and looked at other women's cycle patterns, I realized that every woman's cycle goes through the full moon, new moon, and everything in between over the period of one year. So, generalizing is not going to give us answers. We need something more precise that can be customized for every woman, to explain her unique bleeding pattern.

A few years ago, I would have scoffed at anyone who told me that astrology could provide important answers to deepen our understanding of menstruation. Many of us think of astrology as generalizing zodiac sign characteristics, as it often does in Western astrological interpretation. But Jyotiṣa Śāstra, which is the Indian astrological science, is different; it is the only science where I could find answers that helped me explain the changes in menstrual bleeding patterns and offer methods of predictability, without generalizing all women's cycles.

Jyotiṣa Śāstra is a vast science that is rooted in the study of astronomy, astrology, and the interaction of astrological bodies.

It is highly mathematical, offering precision and predictability. The key differentiating factor between Western astrology and Jyotiṣa Śāstra is that the former is a solar-based system with a movable zodiac, while the latter is a moon or lunar-based system with a fixed zodiac, 27 nakṣatras (lunar constellations), and an assessment based on daśa, which is the period of different planets transiting through different signs and their influence in real-time. Thus, in the Indian system, we see the coming together of astronomy (the study of positions, motions, and properties of celestial bodies) and astrology (the study of how the positions, motions, and properties of celestial bodies influence human beings). This knowledge becomes crucial while studying the celestial influences on the menstrual cycle.

Menstrual patterns

In the context of understanding menstruation, I began by documenting period dates. I have documented my dates for 16 months and also collected the dates of three other women for the purpose of comparative understanding. The following aspects were looked into with the data gathered:

1. Influence of Moon's cycle on menstrual patterns
2. Influence of Sun's cycle on menstrual patterns
3. Influence of other planets on menstrual patterns

I have sought help and guidance from astrologer Annapoorna Bhat ji, who is based in Bengaluru, to study and decode the menstrual dates as per Jyotiṣa Śāstra. What is presented below is by no means a formal comprehensive study. According to Annapoorna ji, it will take at least 200 women with no obvious menstrual disorders, to note down the precise dates and time of the start of menses each month, for about two years, to arrive at conclusive answers. However, the process followed and the observations are still important, as they provide guidelines to understand menstruation from a unique perspective. In the future, formal studies along these lines can be undertaken by those interested.

Influence of the Moon's cycle

Be it in prose or poetry, women have often been compared to the Moon and women's emotional swings to the waxing and waning of the Moon. The reason for this comparison might be more than just creative liberty.

Astronomically speaking, the distance between the Moon and Earth is about 238,855 miles. The Moon completes one rotation around the Earth in 27.32 days approximately. The circumference of the Moon is 6783 miles. One lunar day is about 24 hours and 54 minutes (from moonrise to moonrise). One candra mās (lunar month), from śukla pratipadā (day one after amāvāsyā) to the next amāvāsyā, is of 29 days, 12 hours, 44 minutes, and 2 seconds. This is also known as the synodic month. Whereas, by the parameter of nakṣatra mās (constellation month), the Moon completes a month in 27 days, 7 hours, 43 minutes, and 12 seconds. This is also known as the sidereal month. The duration of nakṣatra mās and the length of a woman's cycle are identical.[1]

The ancient text on Indian astrology, Brihat Jātaka[2], refers to the Sun as the soul and Moon as the mind of the Kālapuruṣa.[3] The Moon is classified as a strī-graha (feminine planet), given that it is the kāraka (significator) for mother and is the ruler of the 4th house (karka/cancer), representing motherly qualities of nurturing. The Moon is said to influence human emotions; as its cycle changes, human emotions have also been observed to undergo changes. In women, these changes manifest in their menstrual cycle patterns.

From my own observations as well as that of other women, when the menstrual date coincides with amāvāsyā (new moon), the menstrual experience comes with greater emotional turmoil than when it coincides with pūrṇimā (full moon). Astrologically, Moon is considered to be strongest at the time of pūrṇimā, since the Earth comes in between the Moon and the Sun at this time. The Moon is weakest at the time of amāvāsyā since it comes between the Earth and Sun at this time, its proximity to the Sun making it weak at this time.

In Āyurved, we say that pūrṇimā is the time when the body's natural immunity is at its peak and there is more ojas, causing menstruation occurring at full moon to be smoother. Whereas amāvāsyā is the time when the body is at its weakest, and consequently, bleeding with amāvāsyā could be an emotionally draining affair. During my work in villages, there have been numerous instances when farmers, even today, take a break on amāvāsyā and refrain from sowing, owing to their experience of plants not growing well if sown during this time. Farmers in India look at the lunar calendar to plan agricultural activity.

If bleeding with amāvāsyā is not the best menstrual experience, then why is it often said to be indicative of good reproductive health?

The answer to this lies in understanding the best times to conceive. Indian sciences consider day 4 (soon after menstruation) up to day 12 (nearing ovulation) as the ideal time to conceive. If women menstruate with amāvāsyā, then conception could occur in śukla pakṣa (waxing phase) and closer to pūrṇimā. This phase is understood to be better for overall health and vitality. Hence, for women in their active reproductive years, bleeding with or close to amāvāsyā is said to be indicative of better health, meaning it is healthier to conceive closer to or during pūrṇimā, after menses in amāvāsyā.

On the other hand, when women are not attempting to conceive or when they are pursuing a spiritual path, their cycles are more useful when it happens closer to or in sync with pūrṇimā. When women bleed with pūrṇimā, the time of amāvāsyā is available to them for sādhana (spiritual practice). This is best explained in the following words of Śrī Amritānanda Nātha Saraswathi, whose biography Goddess and the Guru offers many insights in this direction:

"Amāvāsyā is very sacred. That is when all the kālas of the moon have gone back to the sun. The union of the sun and moon is complete in amāvāsyā. That is when the suṣumṇa channel is active. Passion and vairāgya (detachment) are completely united. That is when the kuṇḍalinī flows through the central channel. The Devī is completely in union with Śiva on amāvāsyā. She is called Kāli. During pūrṇimā, full moon, Devī is completely separate. She is Lalita then."

For those following a spiritual path, the role of suṣumṇa nāḍī is crucial, as it is the key pathway to attain spiritual heights. Activating this suṣumṇa nāḍī is said to be easier during amāvāsyā, making this time of the month significant for the spiritual aspirant.

Influence of the Sun's cycle

The very first sloka of Brihat Jātaka talks of the Sun as that which gives form to the Moon. In a lunar calendar, we keep time by looking at the phases of the Moon. But there is an overarching understanding that it is the Sun that causes these phases of the Moon to occur. As the Sun passes through the solstices[5] and equinox,[6] it causes a shift in our cycle. In India, the Sun's cycle, marked by the solstice, is known as the ayana. Uttarāyaṇa refers to the months between the winter solstice and the summer solstice (approximately Dec 22nd to June 21st), and Dakṣiṇāyana refers to the months between the summer solstice and the winter solstice (approximately June 22nd to Dec 21st). The equinox occurs around March 20th and September 22nd in India.

By plotting dates of menstruation, dates of amāvāsyā, and pūrṇimā, the influence of the ayanas and equinox on the menstrual pattern can be observed. In the given charts, by observing how the line with the period dates intersects the lines with amāvāsyā and pūrṇimā dates, we can observe how the menstrual shifts happen closer to the solstice and equinox.

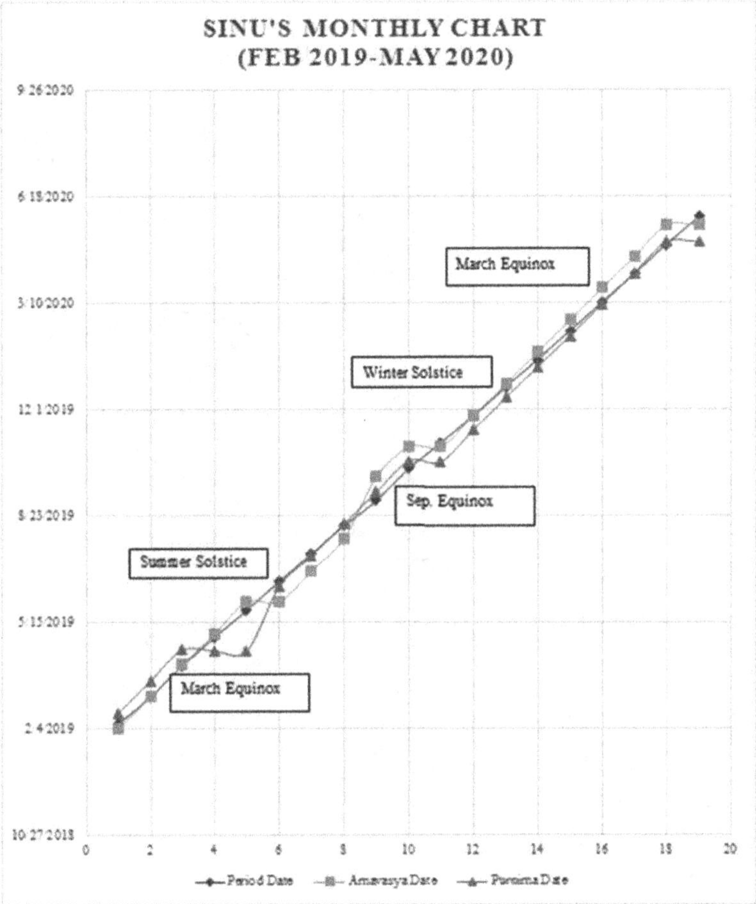
SINU'S MONTHLY CHART
(FEB 2019-MAY 2020)
9/26/2020
6/18/2020
3/10/2020
12/1/2019
8/23/2019
5/15/2019
2/4/2019
10/27/2018
0
2
4
6
8
10
12
14
16
18
20
March Equinox
Winter Solstice
Sep. Equinox
Summer Solstice
March Equinox
Period Date
Amavasya Date
Purnima Date

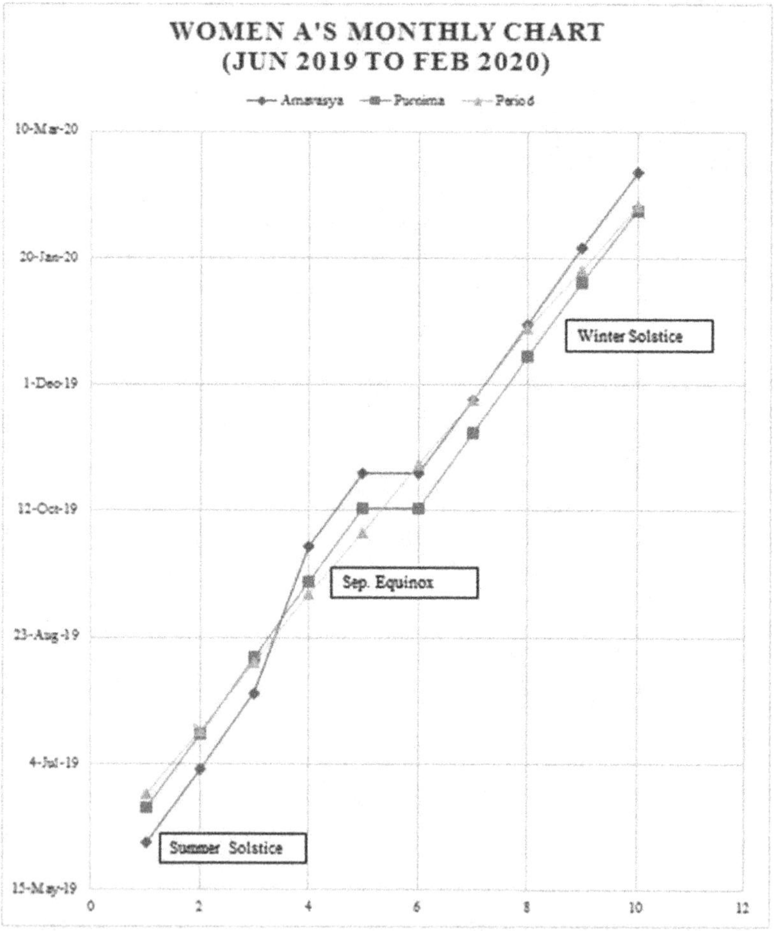
WOMEN A'S MONTHLY CHART
(JUN 2019 TO FEB 2020)
Amavasya
Purnima
Period
10-Mar-20
20-Jan-20
1-Dec-19
12-Oct-19
23-Aug-19
4-Jul-19
15-May-19
0
2
4
6
8
10
12
Winter Solstice
Sep. Equinox
Summer Solstice

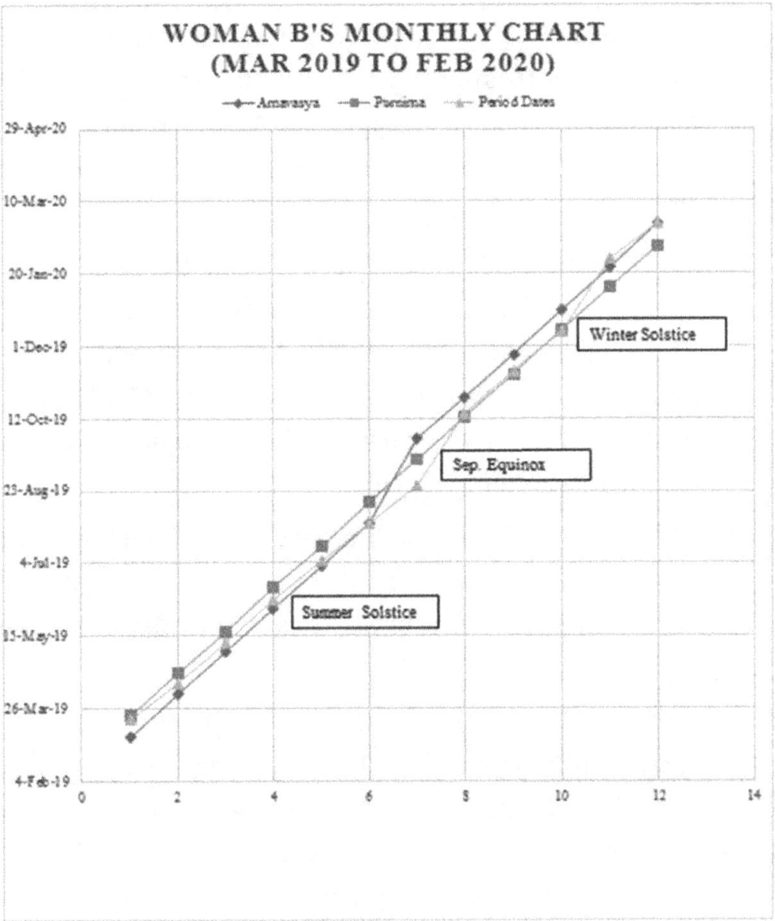
WOMAN B'S MONTHLY CHART
(MAR 2019 TO FEB 2020)
Amavasya
Purnima
Period Dates
29-Apr-20
10-Mar-20
20-Jan-20
1-Dec-19
12-Oct-19
23-Aug-19
4-Jul-19
15-May-19
26-Mar-19
4-Feb-19
0
2
4
6
8
10
12
14
Winter Solstice
Sep. Equinox
Summer Solstice

- The period line is almost straight in my chart and in that of Woman A's chart. Whereas, it is slightly off in the chart of Woman B (in Aug), who reported some disturbances in her cycle at that time.
- In my chart, the period line starts with being close to amāvāsyā (Feb 4th) by occurring on Feb 9th. Then it coincides with amāvāsyā on the menstrual date of 6th March 2019. Post the equinox in March, it continues to occur close to amāvāsyā (April 5th) by occurring on April 4th.
- In the month of May, there were two dates of menses, May 1st and May 26th. The first date occurred close to amāvāsyā (May 4th) and the second was mid-way between pūrṇimā (May 18th) and the next amāvāsyā (June 3rd). Here, we see the shift happening from amāvāsyā to pūrṇimā as we near the summer solstice.
- The next date (June 22nd) moves toward pūrṇimā after the summer solstice on 21st June 2019. In August, the period date (Aug 13th) is very near to pūrṇimā date (Aug 15th).
- As the September equinox nears, the period date shifts away from pūrṇimā (Oct 13th) and starts moving closer to amāvāsyā (Oct 27th) by occurring on Oct 6th and Oct 31st. It coincides with amāvāsyā again in November (Nov 25th) and occurs close to the next amāvāsyā (Dec 25th) by occurring on Dec 22nd. After the winter solstice on 22nd December 2019, it moves toward pūrṇimā again, and the annual pattern alternates.
- Note that if the dates occur around amāvāsyā in Jan 2019, then it will occur around pūrṇimā in Jan 2020,

then again in amāvāsyā in Jan 2021, and so on. By tracing the dates for a period of two years, we will be able to see one complete cycle. A similar two-year pattern will be observed even when we look at it astrologically, as we will see in the next section.

- Woman A's chart is very similar to mine. Woman B's chart also has similar cycles, though a bit delayed.

The chart of an adolescent girl, aged 12, who attained menarche in June 2019 is shown below. Her chart indicates how she started menarche close to amāvāsyā in June 2019 and underwent the shift to pūrṇimā in December 2019, clearly indicating the effect of the solstices. The variations in between are perhaps owing to it being that of an adolescent girl's initial cycles trying to stabilize.

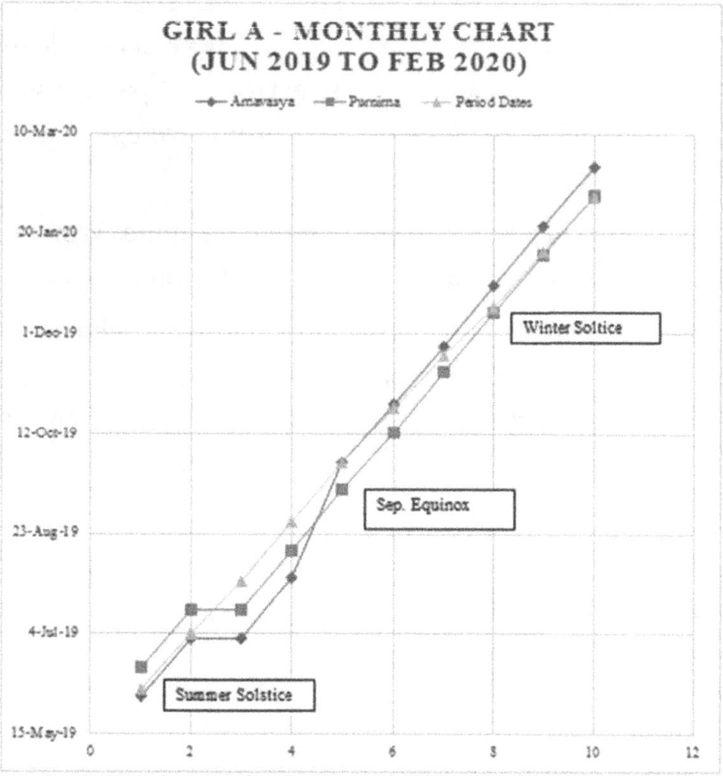

It is important that those who take this up as a formal study should include as many women with healthy cycles and minimal other health issues, in order to see patterns as they should occur. For the purpose of undertaking this work, I was extremely cautious about my health for the duration of this study, with regular practice of yōg āsana, prāṇāyāma, a vegetarian diet, and no other prominent health issues. All women who shared their menstrual dates were in their late thirties.

Influence of other planets

Now is when it gets really interesting. We will now move from generalizations of the Moon and Sun's cycles to specifics of what causes menstruation to occur. For this, the guidance of an experienced astrologer becomes important. To find a learned astrologer who is well versed with ancient science is difficult on its own; to find a woman who is a learned astrologer is like searching for a pin in a haystack. What is presented below could not have been possible without the support of Annapoorna ji, to whom I remain grateful for guiding me in this exercise.

Within the female body, menstruation is the time when pitta is predominant. Pitta is indicative of heat and the energy of transformation. I always wondered whether a similar condition of pitta dominance to cause menses might occur every month due to the influence of any particular planet. And to my surprise, the ancient text Brihat Jātaka, written by Varahamihira (born in 505 AD), talks of the planet Mars (also known as Kuja or Mangal) as the cause for menstruation, along with the Moon.

Mars is the red hot planet whose element is agni (fire) and whose humor is pitta, according to Jyotiṣa Śāstra. Mars rules over blood while the Moon rules over the bodily fluids of women. The coming together of Mars and Moon is said to cause menstruation every month. In Chapter 4, sloka 1 of Brihat Jātaka, the following verses are written. The English translation[6] is also provided.

कुजेन्दुहेतु प्रतिमासमार्तवं गते तु पीडर्क्षमनुण्णदीधितौ ।

अतोन्यथास्थे शुभपुंग्रहेक्षिते नरेण संयोगमुपैति कामिनी ॥ १ ॥

kujenduhetu pratimāsamārtavaṃ gate tu pīḍārkśamanuṇadīdhitau

atonyathāsthe śubhapuṃgraheksịte nareṇa saṃyogamupaiti kāminī

"The menses of a woman which are due to the interaction of Mars and Moon, set in every month when the Moon is in an anupacaya sthāna (1st, 2nd 4th, 5th, 7th, 8th, 9th or 12th house) from the lagna (ascendant). But if the Moon occupies a different position, that is, it is an upacaya sthāna (3rd, 6th, 10th or 11th house) and is aspected by a benefic male planet (meaning Jupiter), the woman lovingly unites with a man."

The meaning of the above sloka will be explained in the following paragraphs, with examples of calculating the menstrual dates and reason for occurrence on that particular date. It is important to note that the above sloka has been written in the context of conception, that is, the dates when women should ideally menstruate in order to have greater chances of a healthy conception.

If you are new to Indian astrology, then it might help that you familiarize yourself with the following basic definitions and terminology before proceeding further. I have only included those definitions which are of relevance in our calculation of menstrual patterns. For more information, the English translation of Brihat Jātaka by V. Subrahmanya Shastri is a good reference.

- **Rāśi** – refers to zodiac sign. The zodiac is a twelve-fold division of the Sun's apparent path along the ecliptic. There are 12 rāśis from Meṣa (Aries) to Mīna (Pisces)[7], similar to that of Western astrology. These are represented by 12 houses in the birth chart. In Jyotiṣa Śāstra, importance is given to the Chandra-Rāśi (moon-sign), that is, the position of the Moon with respect to the rāśi, at the time of birth. The Moon transits the 12 zodiac signs, staying on each one of them for about 2-2.5

days. For menstrual calculation, the chandra-rāśi is considered for each menstrual date.

- **Nakṣatra** - refers to the lunar constellation. There are 27 nakṣatras, each measuring 13.2 degrees (13 degrees and 20 minutes). Each of its parts is called pada. Each pada has the characteristics of a sign of the zodiac, starting with Aries. The Moon spends a little over one day in each nakṣatra. For each menstrual date (with the time of start of menses known), if we note the corresponding nakṣatra, we can observe a particular order of movement, month after month.
- **Graha** - refers to the planet. In Jyotiṣa Śāstra, the 12 zodiac signs are considered as relatively fixed, while the grahas are the moving bodies in the backdrop of the nakṣatras. Only nine grahas are taken into account, viz., Sun, Moon, Mars, Mercury, Jupiter, Venus, Saturn, and Rahu and Ketu (north and south nodes of the moon) respectively. Uranus, Neptune, and Pluto are not visible to the naked eye and are not considered in Jyotiṣa Śāstra.
- **Lagna** - refers to the ascendant. The ascendant is the point on the eastern horizon of the sky at the moment of birth. In a chart, the ascendant represents the body and intelligence, the Moon the emotions and mental faculty, and the Sun the soul of the individual.
- **Anupacaya and Upacaya** - Anupacaya refers to houses numbering 1, 2, 4, 5, 7, 8, 9, 12. The remaining houses, viz., 3, 6, 19, 11, are called upacaya houses.
- **Hora** - refers to an hour. On each of the seven days of a week, starting from the sunrise or sunset time, there are

24 horas ruled by the seven planets. So, each planet could have 2 or 3 horas in a day. Hora is used to determine the exact hour during which a particular planet's effect is dominant. For studying the occurrence of menstruation, we need to look at the hora of Mars since it coincides with the time when menses will begin each month.

- **Gochara** – refers to the transit of planets. The gochara of Mars and Moon is considered for each menstrual date.
- **Aspect** – refers to the angle that planets make to each other. If Mars aspects Moon in its 4th, 7th, or 8th house, it indicates that menses could occur. When planets are in the same house, it is called a conjunction.

With this basic information, we may now proceed to understand in more detail the menstrual patterns and observation as per Jyotiṣa Śāstra. In order to calculate if menstrual dates documented are occurring as it should, the following steps were undertaken:

Step 1: The birth chart of the woman under consideration was prepared with the help of the astrologer. A reliable software can also be used. This requires the woman's exact time of birth, date of birth, and location (latitude and longitude) of birth. Refer to the below chart for Woman A. As per Jyotiṣa Śāstra, the rāśi (zodiac) is fixed and numbered 1 to 12, with 1 indicating Meṣa (Aries) and 12 indicating Mīna (Pisces). The positions of the nine planets at the time of birth are also shown in each house.

12	1	2	3 Ra
11			4
10 **Mo** **Lagna** (Ascendent)	Woman A's Rāśi Chart		5
9 Ma Ke	8 Su Me Ve	7 Ju Sa	6

(In the above chart, Mo = Moon, Ma = Mars, Ke = Ketu, Su = Sun, Me = Mercury, Ve = Venus, Ju = Jupiter, Sa = Saturn, Ra = Rahu)

Step 2: From the birth chart above, the position of the Moon (in house no. 10) is noted. This becomes house no. 1 while counting the anupacaya and upacaya houses for menstrual date validation. Anupacaya houses (1st, 2nd, 4th, 5th, 7th, 8th, 9th, 12th) are colored in the below representation. This indicates that the Moon, during its transit, should be in any of the anupacaya sthānas for menses to occur (leading to successful conception post menses).

<table>
<tr><td>3
Mīna</td><td>4
Meṣa</td><td>5
Vṛṣabha</td><td>6
Mithuna</td></tr>
<tr><td>2
Kumbha</td><td rowspan="2" colspan="2">Woman A
Moon Anupacaya Sthāna</td><td>7
Karka</td></tr>
<tr><td>1
Mo
Makara</td><td>8
Simha</td></tr>
<tr><td>12
Dhanu</td><td>11
Vṛścika</td><td>10
Tula</td><td>9
Kanya</td></tr>
</table>

Step 3: For each date of menstruation, we check if it is occurring in a chandra-rāśi (moon zodiac) which is in an anupacaya house. If yes, then the date is correct. For example, in Woman A's chart below, 22nd June 2019 occurs during the transit of Moon in the zodiac of Kumbha (Aquarius), which is in the anupacaya house 2 and therefore correct. Whereas, 3rd October 2019 occurs in the Vṛścika rāśi (Scorpio), which is in the upacaya house 11 and therefore not a good date with respect to conception post menses. The chandra rāśi of each date can be checked with the help of the astrologer or through a reliable software/website.

Step 4: If the menstrual date is in an anupacaya sthāna, next check if there is any co-relation between Mars and Moon on that day. This means, one or more of the following criteria needs to be satisfied.

a. If there is a hora (specific hour) of Mars transit at the time when menses started on that date

b. If Mars and Moon are in conjunction (same house) on that date

c. If Mars aspects Moon on 4th, 7th, and 8th houses from itself. This should be checked in the gochara (transit) of Mars and Moon for the specific date

d. If it is a Tuesday (Mangalwar), influence of Mars will be there

e. If the rāśi (zodiac) has Mars as its ruler, such as Meṣa/Aries or Vṛścika/Scorpio, the influence of Mars will be there

A table with the information of each date for Woman A is presented below. This information would be more accurate if women note down the start time of menses each month, as the moon remains in one rāśi for about 2.5 days and about 2.3 days in one nakṣatra. Woman A reported her menses as occurring during the day. Therefore, her rāśi, nakṣatra, and hora were calculated accordingly for her location, which is in Coimbatore, Tamil Nadu, India.

Table 6: Woman A's menstrual date analysis

Menstrual Dates	Chandra Rāśi	Nakṣatra & their Order	House	Analysis
22-Jun-2019	Kumbha/ Aquarius	Dhaniṣṭha (23)	Anupacaya house 2	Moon is in an anupacaya sthāna. There is Mars' hora from 8:11 am to 9:14 am. Therefore, the date is correct.
17-July-2019	Makara/ Capricorn	Uttara Āṣāḍha (21)	Anupacaya house 1	Moon is in an anupacaya sthāna. There is Mars' hora from 10:22 am to 11:25 am. Also, Mars aspects Moon in the 7th house. Therefore, the date is correct.
13-Aug-2019	Dhanu/ Saggitarius	Śrāvaṇa (22)	Anupacaya house 12	Moon is in an anupacaya sthāna. There is Mars' hora from 06:15 am to 07:17 am. Also, being a Tuesday, the influence of Mars is there. Therefore, the date is correct.
9-Sep-2019	Dhanu	Uttara Āṣāḍha (21)	Anupacaya house 12	Moon is in an anupacaya sthāna. There is Mars' hora from 09:17 am to 10:18 am. Therefore, the date is correct.
3-Oct-2019	Vṛścika	Anūrādha (17)	Upacaya house 11	Moon is in an upacaya sthāna, making it an incorrect date. However, there is Mars' hora from 7:13 am to 8:13 am, making menses possible at that time.

Menstrual Dates	Chandra Rāśi	Nakṣatra & their Order	House	Analysis
30-Oct 2019	Vṛścika	Anūrādha (17)	Upacaya house 11	Moon is in an upacaya sthāna, making it an incorrect date. However, there is Mars' hora from 10:09 am to 11:07 am, making menses possible at that time.
25-Nov-2019	Tula	Svāti (15)	Upacaya house 10	Moon is in an upacaya sthāna, making it an incorrect date. However, there is Mars' hora from 9:17 am to 10:17 am.
23-Dec-2019	Tula	Viśākha (16)	Upacaya house 10	Moon is in an upacaya sthāna, making it an incorrect date. However, Moon and Mars are conjunct on this date, thereby influencing menses.
15-Jan-2020	Simha	Uttara Phālgunī (12)	Anupacaya house 8	Moon is in an anupacaya sthāna. There is Mars' hora from 10:37 am to 11:34 am.
10-Feb-2020	Simha	Māgha (10)	Anupacaya 8	Moon is in an anupacaya sthāna. There is Mars' hora from 9:42 am to 10:40 am.

Step 5: Prepare a chart with the menstrual dates as per the given criteria. Woman A's monthly menstrual chart will look as below. The menstrual charts of two more women are given below for comparison.

3 Mīna	4 Meṣa	5 Vṛṣabha	6 Mithuna
2 22-Jun-2019 Kumbha	Woman A's Monthly Menses Dates (Jun 2019 to Feb 2019)		7 Karka
1 17-Jul-2019 Mo Makara			8 15-Jan-2020 10-Feb-2020 Simha
12 13-Aug-2019 9-Sep-2019 Dhanu	11 3-Oct-2019 30-Oct-2019 Vṛścika	10 25-Nov-2019 23-Dec-2019 Tula	9 Kanya

7 9-Feb-2019 4-Apr-2019 1-May-2019 Mīna	8 Meṣa	9 Vṛṣabha	10 Mithuna
6 6-Mar-2019 26-May-2019 Kumbha	Sinu's Monthly Menses Dates (Feb 2019 to May 2020)		11 Karka
5 21-Jun- 2019 18-Jul-2019 Makara			12 6-Apr-2020 Simha
4 13-Aug-2019 6-Oct-2019 Dhanu	3 6-Sep-2019 31-Oct-2019 Vṛścika	2 25-Nov-2019 22-Dec-2019 Tula	1 11-Mar-2020 13-Feb-2020 17-Jan-2020 Mo Kanya

5 30-Jan-2020 Mīna	6 15-Oct-2019 Meṣa	7 14-Nov-2019 11-Dec-2019 Vṛṣabha	8 12-Apr-2019 10-May-2019 26-Aug-2019 Mithuna
4 24-Feb-2020 Kumbha	Woman B's Monthly Menses Dates (Mar 2019 to Feb 2020)		9 1-Aug-2019 Karka
3 Makara			10 19-Mar-2019 9-Jun-2019 6-Jul-2019 Simha
2 Dhanu	1 Mo Vṛścika	12 Tula	11 Kanya

Observations

- In all the charts above, we can see that the dates occupy one-half of the chart. In the case of Woman A and myself, it is the left half of the chart. In the case of Woman B, it is the right half. This indicates cyclicity and also the fact that it takes two years to complete one full chart. This means the menstrual dates cover all rāśis in two years, in a specific order, barring a few outliers.
- Even if we note only the nakṣatras, we can see the same pattern of moving in a particular order. This can be seen in the tabular column of Woman A's menstrual dates when it moves in descending order from nakṣatra numbered 23 to

10 (barring a few outliers). Here again, it takes two years for the monthly menses dates to cover all 27 nakṣatras.

- All three charts have four dates which occur in the upacaya sthāna. When Moon is in the upacaya sthāna during menses, it indicates that those particular months are not ideal for conception post menses.

When our cycles are completely out of sync, it will usually be found to be moving up and down 2-3 rāśis, instead of progressing in a cyclical way through each rāśi. When this pattern was observed in the cycle of one particular woman (see Woman D's chart below), I enquired if she had any menstrual problems. She said that her period was fine and occurred every month. However, upon deeper inquiry, I learned that she was going through stressful times.

10 Mīna	11 Meṣa	12 Vṛṣabha	1 Mo Mithuna
9 24-Dec-2017 19-Jan-2018 Kumbha	Woman D's Monthly Menses Dates (Jan 2017 to Jan 2018)		2 Karka
8 Makara			3 Simha
7 21-Feb-2017 10-Jun-2017 07-Jul-2017 25-Oct-2017 23-Nov-2017 Dhanus	6 24-Jan-2017 19-Mar-2017 13-May-2017 03-Aug-2017 30-Aug-2017 25-Sep-2017 Vṛścika	5 13-04-2017 Tula	4 Kanya

Like her, many women consider their cycle to be alright if it shows up every month. But when we chart it astrologically, we will begin to see patterns that can be early signs of a future problem. Remember, the Moon is indicative of the mind and emotions. Therefore, emotional stress will be the first to show up in the chart, before it manifests as menstrual issues.

Conclusion

Some of you may feel that the above information is too complex owing to the unfamiliarity with astrology and the calculations involved. That is understandable. The least you can take home is that women's menstrual cycles have patterns. This means we can look at simpler signs each month to know if our period is progressing as it should and if there are any factors, such as stress, causing changes in the pattern. To begin with, we can start noting down the date and time of the start of menses each month. One of the interesting things to note is that the start of bleeding each month occurs during the hour (hora) when there is the influence of Mars in your location. This can be checked with a location-specific daily hora chart. We can also observe the pattern of the dates with respect to the phases of the Moon and the cycles of the Sun, and see how it repeats every two years. Further, with the help of an astrologer or by using the method prescribed above, we can look at more precise details as per Jyotiṣa Śāstra. Once familiar with these methods, it is possible to even predict the menstrual date each month with reasonable accuracy.

Rural women in India tend to observe their cycles as a matter of habit. Not only do they observe their cycles, but they also observe how it impacts their overall health and are quick to pick up deviations from the norm. For them, as it should be for us, menstrual cycles are more than an indicator of reproductive ability. Our monthly period dates are our wellness indicators. All we need to do is learn how to read it.

References for Chapter 6

1. Chandrashekar Sharma. www.jyotishteaching.com, 2008.
2. Brihat Jataka by Varahamihira. Chapter 2, Sloka 1.
3. In Indian Astrology, the zodiac is represented by the body of the Kalapurusha
4. Solstice - The day that the Earth's North Pole is tilted closest to the Sun is called Summer Solstice. It is the day when the Sun reaches its highest point in the sky, resulting in the longest day in the year. The Winter Solstice, which is the shortest day in the year, happens when the Earth's North Pole is tilted farthest from the Sun. In the Northern Hemisphere (India), June marks the Summer Solstice. This is reversed for the Southern Hemisphere.
5. Equinox refers to the day when the Sun is exactly above the equator, making the length of the day and night to become equal.
6. Shastri, Subrahmanya V. Brihat Jataka English Translation, 2nd edition. 1956. Chapter 4, sloka 1.
7. Aries (Meṣa), Taurus (Vṛṣabha), Gemini (Mithuna), Cancer (Karka), Leo (Simha), Virgo (Kanya), Libra (Tula), Scorpio (Vṛścika), Sagittarius (Dhanu), Capricorn (Makara), Aquarius (Kumbha), Pisces (Mīna).

CHAPTER 7

GIFTS OF THE MENSTRUAL CYCLE

Women in the menstruating age sometimes consider themselves to be at a disadvantage compared to men. Menstruation, for a number of women, is at best an inconvenience to be tolerated. Women feel that menstruation comes in the way of being productive and equal to men. But the fact is that this very aspect of menstruation gives women a decisive advantage—not only because menstruation cleanses the inner system and maintains overall health, but also because the entire menstrual cycle offers a unique opportunity month after month to start afresh, physically and emotionally. This knowledge can greatly enhance women's productivity at work, their outlook on life, and help to deal with stressful situations with the least turmoil.

Doṣas not only influence the few days of menstruation but also the entire monthly menstrual cycle, known as ṛtu cakra. Modern medicine provides some information on the menstrual phases, with respect to hormones. But hormones are influenced by the doṣas. So, understanding both doṣas and hormones during each phase of the menstrual cycle is a great way to know what is happening within our body. During each week of the menstrual cycle, a particular doṣa is predominant. Being aware of this each week can help women plan their work better and make the most of nature's gift.

1. Rajah-srāva-kāla (menstrual phase) – Days 1 to 4 (sometimes, up to 7)

Modern medicine observes that the hormones estrogen and progesterone are at an all-time low during menstruation. Often, this low level of hormones is attributed to the lack of physical energy and feeling of exhaustion experienced at the time of menstruation.

According to Āyurved, rajah srāva kāla is mainly influenced by vāta. It is well known that the movement of any substance from one place to another is the function of vāta doṣa. Menstrual flow is considered to be a function of the subtype of vāta called apāna.[1] Vāta doṣa is predominant during menstruation, and consequently, the duration of menstrual flow is characterized by vāta, physically and emotionally. When the menstrual cycle is healthy, the same phase can become a time of inward contemplation, inner cleansing, and strong intuition guiding women to make important changes in life. Often, new creative ideas emerge forth at this time, as vāta is responsible for all creative pursuits. For me, even the idea of writing this book surfaced on a menstrual day.

With menstruation, every month, women are offered a chance to start afresh and press the reset button. It is an opportunity to let go of whatever is not working for us and prepare to begin a new chapter. This is the time when the body longs to become still and our inner voice will begin to be heard. The practice of menstrual leave is a great way to tune in to this inner wisdom and creativity. When women are in good physical and emotional health, menstruation can be similar to a sādhana (spiritual practice) in itself.

2. Ṛtu-kāla (proliferative phase including ovulation) – Days 4 to 12

The hormone estrogen begins to rise about ten days after menstruation and reaches its peak at ovulation. Estrogen causes thickening of the endometrium lining in preparation for pregnancy and is said to be responsible for increased energy levels and stamina in women. There is also a rise in testosterone at this time, although much lesser than what is produced in men. Testosterone is considered to cause an increase in sexual libido and increased muscular strength for women.

As per Āyurved, the process of rebuilding the endometrium could mean that there is a dominance of kapha doṣa in this phase.[1] This phase starts just after menstruation and goes up to the time of ovulation. At this time, women are at their energetic best, physically, and feel more stable, emotionally. There are fewer emotional upheavals at this time, and women will have better endurance and strength during the week after menstruation. The immunity that kapha doṣa brings reflects in the glow of the skin, post menstruation. For women, this is the ideal time to plan physical work, outdoor activity, or take on a challenging task. In terms of work, women will have greater stamina and the ability to push working hours at this time.

Āyurved also recommends this phase as the ideal phase for conceiving a child. Kapha improves fertility in women and enhances the natural immune system, making it an ideal time to conceive.

3. Ṛtu vyatīta kāla (secretory phase)

As per modern medicine, there will be a rise in progesterone levels soon after ovulation. Progesterone maintains the thickness of the endometrium lining. When progesterone levels drop around the 28th day, the endometrium sheds its lining along with the unfertilized egg, resulting in what we call menstruation. The rise in progesterone is said to be responsible for pre-menstrual symptoms (PMS).

Note that period postponing pills contain synthetic progesterone, which artificially keeps progesterone levels high and prevents endometrium shedding, thereby delaying menstruation. Those who take such pills will experience PMS-like symptoms. Such synthetic hormones can play havoc with the sensitive menstrual cycle, causing internal confusion, and are best to be avoided.

In Āyurved, during ṛtu vyatīta kāla, the function of dhatvāgni is increased. Agni is the pañcabhautika constituent of pitta. Hence, it can be said that this phase is influenced by pitta doṣa.[1] During this phase, pitta doṣa begins to rise to aid the transformative process of ovulation. Pitta brings with it the qualities of passion, drive, and sexual desire manifesting during ovulation. Women tend to become more aware of their sexuality at this time. As the date nears menstruation, some women may feel an increased capacity to work due to the dominance of pitta. However, it will also cause them to feel exhausted soon. The predominance of pitta doṣa just before menstruation results in pre-menstrual symptoms or PMS, such as increased hunger and thirst, body heat, acne, physical exhaustion, etc. When pitta is aggravated, sudden bursts of anger are an indication that menstruation is nearing.

If we slow down at this time and become observant of the changes that happen just before menstruation, we will notice that this is the most revealing phase, wherein all that is not working for us becomes obvious and clear. The mask of diplomacy is lifted. The clarity in thought, emboldened by the fire of pitta, means that women in this phase end up confronting things that are diplomatically pushed under the carpet at other times. This is the time when women no longer feel the need to fit into others' definition of what they should be, and instead become bold enough to live life by their own rules. Consequently, major changes in relationships and work could manifest at this time. Unfortunately, modern women are taught to suppress these intuitive feelings and act 'normal' or else be ridiculed as PMSing. If women learn to trust what their PMS time is telling them, they will make large strides in life and avoid prolonged emotional suffering.

Earth's fertility cycle

In India, we refer to the earth as Mother Earth or Mother Nature. She is feminine; we have no doubt about that. Women in India are believed to be a manifestation of the Great Mother herself. This is not just symbolic. In India, the six seasons and their shifts follow the same phases as a woman's menstrual cycle. Just as the doṣas within the female body change every week, bringing them unique gifts, so also the doṣas within Mother Earth's body change every season, resembling a woman's menstrual and fertility cycle. According to the changes in the season, our diet, lifestyle, and exercise routine need to change. In Āyurved, this knowledge is called ṛtucārya—the daily regimen to be followed, keeping in mind the seasonal changes.

The year, according to Āyurved, is divided into two periods depending on the direction of movement of Sun, that is, uttarāyaṇa (northern solstice), also known as ādāna kāla and dakṣiṇāyana (southern solstice), also known as visarga kāla. Each is formed of three ṛtu (seasons). The word ṛtu is also one of the Saṃskṛtam names for menstruation, indicating the close connection between the seasonal changes on Earth and in a woman's menstrual cycle. The seasons in uttarāyaṇa are śiśira (winter), vasanta (spring), and grīṣma (summer), while the seasons in dakṣiṇāyana are varṣā (monsoon), śaradā (autumn), and hemanta (late autumn).[8] Each season has an inherent dominance of one or more mahābhūtas, causing aggravation or pacification of specific doṣas. The regimen prescribed under Ṛtu-cārya aims to enhance the opposite qualities in a given season, so as to neutralize the tendency of doṣa vitiation in that season and thereby prevent disease.

The table below summarizes the seasons, the predominant pañcamāhabhūta and rasa associated with each season, the impact on the human body, and the regimen to be followed as per Ṛtucārya practices from Suśruta saṃhita and Caraka saṃhita[2, 3].

Table 7: Ṛtu-cārya as per seasons

Seasons & months	Predominant Mahābhūta & Rasa	Effect on humans	Ṛtu-cārya - Regimen prescribed
Śiśira/ Winter Mid-Jan to Mid-Feb	Mahābhūta: ākāśa (ether) Rasa: Tikta (bitter)	✦ The cold, dry effect of vāta is predominant. ✦ Accumulated Kapha from last season (hemanta) will cause problems such as sinusitis and congestion, for some. ✦ Strength is less, there is deposition of kapha doṣa. The abdominal fire becomes dull owing to the internal cold and dries up the bodily rasa.	✦ Diet: Food items having amla (sour) as the predominant taste is preferred. Cereals and pulses, wheat/gram flour products, new rice, corn are advised. Ginger, garlic, haritakī (fruits of Terminalia chebula), pippalī (fruits of Piper longum), sugarcane products, milk, and milk products are to be included in the diet. ✦ Foods having kaṭu (pungent), tikta (bitter), kaṣāya (astringent) predominant rasa are to be avoided. Laghu (light) and śīta (cold) foods are advised to be prohibited. ✦ Massage with oil/powder/paste, bathing with lukewarm water, exposure to sunlight, wearing warm clothes are to be followed. ✦ Vāta aggravating lifestyle like exposure to cold wind, excessive walking, sleeping late at night, etc. are to be avoided.
Vasanta/ Spring Mid-Mar to Mid-May	Mahābhūta: pṛthvī (earth), vāyu (air) Rasa: kaṣāya (astringent)	✦ The bodily Kapha already stored in the body owing to the coldness of the body during the hemanta season is aggravated during the spring by the (increasing) heat (of the sun and consequently of the organism) and could give rise to many diseases. ✦ Strength of the person remains in medium degree, vitiation of Kapha Doṣa occurs, and agni remains in manda (dull) state.	✦ One should take easily digestible food. Among cereals, old barley, wheat, rice are preferred. Among pulses, lentil, mugda (mūng bean) can be taken. Food items tasting tikta (bitter), kaṭu (pungent), and kaṣāya (astringent) are to be taken. Besides those, honey is to be included in the diet. ✦ Food which are hard to digest are to be avoided. Those which are śīta (cold), snigdha (viscous), guru (heavy), amla (sour), madhura (sweet) are not preferred. New grains, curd, cold drinks, and so on are also prohibited. ✦ One should use warm water for bathing & may exercise during Vasant Ṛtu. Udvartana (massage) with powder of candana (Santalum album), kesara (Crocus sativus), and others, kavala (gargle), dhūma (smoking), āñjana (collyrium), and evacuative measures such as vamana (emetic) and nasya (medicinal powder to be inhaled) are advised. ✦ Day-sleep is strictly contraindicated during this season. ✦ Sexual pleasure may be enjoyed in this season.

Seasons & months	Predominant Mahābhūta & Rasa	Effect on humans	Ṛtu-cārya - Regimen prescribed
Grīṣma/ Summer Mid-May to Mid-July	Mahābhūta: agni (fire) & vāyu (air) Rasa: kaṭu (pungent)	✦ The strength of the person becomes less, deposition of Vāta Doṣa occurs, but the vitiated Kapha Doṣa is pacified during this season.	✦ Sweet-scented and cooling pānaka and manthā (types of beverage) with an abundance of sugar should be used. ✦ Foods that are light to digest—those having madhura (sweet), snigdha (unctuous), śīta (cold), and drava (liquid), such as rice, lentil, etc., are to be taken. ✦ Lavaṇa (salt) and food with kaṭu (pungent) and amla (sour) taste and uṣṇa (heat inducing) foods are to be avoided. ✦ Staying in cool places, applying sandalwood and other aromatic pastes over the body, adorning with flowers, wearing light clothes, and sleeping at daytime are helpful. At night, one can enjoy the cool moon rays and evening breeze. ✦ Physical exercise, toil, hot and excessively drying articles should be avoided. ✦ Excessive sexual indulgence and alcoholic preparations are prohibited in this season.
Varṣā/ Monsoon Mid-July to Mid-Sep	Mahābhūta: pṛthvī (earth) & agni (fire) Rasa: amla (sour)	✦ The bodily vāyu of a person is generally aggravated during the varṣā season owing to a slimy condition of the organism, producing impairment of the digestive fire as well as goose-flesh on the skin. ✦ The strength of the person again becomes less, vitiation of vāta doṣa and deposition of pitta doṣa occur. ✦ Agni also gets vitiated.	✦ The herbs and vegetables being newly grown in this (rainy) season are (over-juicy and) consequently not very easy to digest. ✦ Articles of astringent, bitter, and pungent tastes should be prescribed for mitigating the aggravation of the bodily doṣas. ✦ The food should be non-liquid and made neither too emollient (fatty or lardacious) nor too rūkṣa (hard or dry), and should be composed of articles which are appetizing and heat-making in their potency. ✦ Water should be boiled and cooled before consumption and can be taken in combination with honey. ✦ The excessive use of physical exercise, water, dew, sexual intercourse, and the sun's rays (which might lead to indigestion) are to be avoided in this season. ✦ Sleep at daytime and eating before the previous meal is digested should be strictly avoided in this season.

(Contd.)

Seasons & months	Predominant Mahābhūta & Rasa	Effect on humans	Ṛtu-cārya - Regimen prescribed
Śaradā/ Autumn Mid-Sep to Mid-Nov	Mahābhūta: āpā (water) & agni (fire) Rasa: Lavaṇa (salty)	✦ The strength of the person remains medium, pacification of vitiated vāta doṣa and vitiation of pitta doṣa occur, and activity of agni increases during this season. ✦ All pitta-subsiding measures should be taken in this season.	✦ Articles of astringent, sweet, and bitter tastes, different preparations of milk and sugarcane juice as well as honey, śāli-rice, mudga-pulse (mūng bean), oil, and the meat of jāṅgala animals (flesh of animals of dry land) should be used in Śaradā ṛtu. ✦ Tīkṣṇa (sharp potencied or pungent), acid, hot and alkaline articles (of food) as well as the sun's rays, sexual excess, sleep at daytime, and keeping late hours should be avoided. ✦ Habit of eating food only when there is a feeling of hunger is recommended. One should take water purified by the rays of sun in daytime and rays of moon at nighttime for drinking, bathing, etc. Clean and thin clothes scented with sandal-pastes or with camphor as well as garlands of autumnal flowers should be worn.
Hemanta/ Late Autumn Mid-Nov to Mid-Jan	Mahābhūta: pṛthvi (earth) & āpā (water) Rasa : madhura (sweet)	✦ The strength of a person remains on highest grade and vitiated pitta doṣa gets pacified. ✦ Activity of agni is increased.	✦ The use of saline, alkaline, bitter, acid, and pungent articles of diet (prepared) with the addition of clarified butter or oil are beneficial. Food should not be taken cold, and drinks prepared with tīkṣṇa (hot potencied) articles (such as strong wine) should be taken, after pasting the body all over with aguru-pastes. ✦ Baths should be taken in tepid water after rubbing in oil all over the body. Large inner apartments completely surrounded by rooms on all sides and containing firepots (serving the purpose of chimneys) should be used as bedrooms, and the bedsheets should be silken. Sufficiently warm coverings for the body should be used. ✦ Sexual indulgence with one partner and residing in warm places are recommended. ✦ Food should not be taken cold, and heating drinks such as strong wines can be taken in this season.

Changes in bala

The Ṛtucārya practices provide us beautiful insights into the lifestyle of our ancestors and help us visualize the way in which ancient Indian society lived in tune with Mother Nature and her cyclical changes, in order to prevent diseases from occurring due to the change in seasons. These practices prescribed the diet and lifestyle regime suitable for each season. An interesting randomized survey study was undertaken (Jangid et al, 2009) to evaluate the effect of ṛtu on bala[4] (strength of an individual) as mentioned in Caraka Suthrasthāna.[5] In the study, 85 healthy volunteers were observed during the hemanta (late autumn), vasanta (spring), and varṣā (rainy) ṛtu (season). The results showed that maximum bala was found in the hemanta ṛtu, moderate bala in the vasanta ṛtu, and minimum or least bala in the varṣā ṛtu.

If we looked at this as per the solstice, we find that at the beginning of visarga kāla (southern solstice) and ending of ādāna kāla (northern solstice), that is, during grīṣma (summer) and varṣā (rainy) seasons, bala is at the lowest. In the middle of the solstices, that is, during śaradā (autumn) and vasanta (spring), bala remains in moderate grade, and at the end of visarga kāla and the beginning of ādāna kāla, that is, during hemanta (late autumn) and śiśira (winter), maximum bala is seen.[6] This bears a wonderful resemblance to the ṛtu cakra or menstrual cycle of a woman.

Mother Earth's menstrual cycle

Observe how the grīṣma (summer) season has a dominance of vāyu and agni, and thereby qualities of vāta and pitta doṣa, resembling the menstrual days of a woman. The regulations on exercise, diet, and even sexual indulgence are similar to what is prescribed for a menstruating woman. Indeed, this is the time when Mother Earth is considered to be menstruating.

In Eastern India's state of Assam, the Ambubachi festival marks the menstruation of Devī Kāmākhya, which is celebrated for four days, starting from the 7th to 11th day of ashada (lunar month in June) and usually happens from June 22nd to June 26th (observe how it starts a day after the summer solstice on June 21st). Similarly, in the state of Odisha, the Raja Parbha festival is celebrated to mark Mother Earth's menstruation in June. People in these states take time off for 3-4 days to acknowledge and celebrate Mother Earth's menstruation. During these 3-4 days, people do not dig the earth and avoid touching/stepping on it as far as possible. Mother Earth is allowed to rest when she menstruates, just like we women are told to rest when we menstruate.

In the South Indian states, at the onset of the lunar month of āṣāḍha in June, married couples are separated, and the wife is sent to her mother's house. This is to prevent the conception of a child in this season, given that there is high vāta and pitta doṣa at this time, resembling the infertile time of menstruation.

Mother Earth's fertile period

Observe the hemanta (late autumn) season, when bala is said to be maximum. At this time, pṛthvī (earth) & āpā (water) are predominant, indicating the qualities of kapha doṣa, making it similar to the ṛtu kāla or proliferative phase of the menstrual cycle. This also makes it the ideal time to conceive. Consequently, sexual indulgence is recommended at this time because the human body is at its strongest at this time, owing to kapha. This is very similar to the fertile days recommended to a woman within her monthly menstrual cycle. It is not a coincidence that this season is considered auspicious for marriages in India. [7]

Thus, we see that a woman's menstrual cycle is similar to that of Mother Earth's cycle, with the grīṣma (summer) season resembling the menstrual phase when bala is the lowest and hemanta (late autumn) season resembling the fertile/ovulatory phase when bala is the highest. Many of the festivals and cultural practices in India associated with seasonal changes arise from this knowledge and are aimed at helping humans align themselves with Mother Earth's cycles.

Being feminine, like nature

For too long, we have confused being a feminist with being feminine. The two are vastly different. Feminism often expects women to operate from a place of utter weakness and helplessness because of the way in which we believe that someone else holds power over women. Women's rights movements are often centered around asking others to give women their power. Distorted versions of such a thought process are what result in FDA approved drugs such as Lybrel that suppress menstruation because it is considered as a deviation from the 'normal' bodily process of a non-menstruating body. It is an insult to the immense potential of what women can offer to the world and the role of the feminine. When we look down upon women, we look down upon Mother Earth, inviting Her wrath.

Being feminine, on the other hand, is when women operate from a place of deep inner knowing and the power that comes from being in a position to give to others, just like

Mother Earth. When women operate from such a space, they become nurturers, doers, social leaders, and default decision-makers, who the community naturally respects and looks up to. In matriarchal societies, women's cycles paved the way for scheduling day-to-day activities. When women menstruated, all activity ceased, including farming. Women's menstrual leaves became the time when everyone rested. This is because it was understood that all subtle processes that happen in nature and among human beings are manifested in obvious ways in a women's body. Respecting a woman's cycle and following its phases was understood to be the most sensible and healthy way of living.

Women's menstrual cycles grant them the gift of knowing, and therefore, of guiding, society at large. When women realize the gifts of their menstrual cycle, the entire human race will shift to a more purposeful and healthier lifestyle which is in sync with Mother Earth's cycles. Nobody else can give women this power; it is already inherent in every woman, waiting to be realized.

References for Chapter 7

1. Dr. Mrs. Arankalle Pournima Sandip. Stri-sharira in classics of Ayurveda: A Critical Review. Scholars Journal of Applied Medical Sciences (SJAMS), Sch. J. App. Med. Sci., 2014; 2(2D):876-881
2. Thakkar J, Chaudhari S, Sarkar PK. Ritucharya: Answer to the lifestyle disorders. Ayu. 2011;32(4):466-471.
3. Kunjlal, Kaviraj. Suśruta Saṃhitā. Uttara Tantra.
4. In Āyurved, bala is not just physical strength, but has a much broader dimension. It refers to the total strength of a human body, at the physical as well as psychological level.
5. Jangid C, Vyas HA, Dwivedi RR. Concept of Ritus and their effect on Bala. AYU Int Res J Ayurveda. 2009;30:11–5
6. Rao Mangalagowri V, editor. Text Book of Svasthavritta. Varanasi: Chaukhamba Orientalia; 2007.
7. Aṣṭāṅgahṛdaya sūtrasthāna prescribes the following regimen for frequency of sexual intercourse - During hemanta (late autumn) and śiśira (winter) the person can indulge in copulation (daily) as much as he likes after making use of aphrodisiacs (and obtaining strength); Once in three days in vasanta (spring) and Śaradā (autumn) and once a fortnight in grīṣma (summer) and varṣā (rainy).
8. Thakkar J, Chaudhari S, Sarkar PK. Ritucharya: Answer to the lifestyle disorders. Ayu. 2011;32(4):466-471. doi:10.4103/0974-8520.96117

PART II
MENSTRUATION IN RELIGION

विद्या समस्तास्तव देवी भेदाः
स्त्रियः समस्तासकला जगत्सु

Vidyā samastāstava devī bhedāh,

Stryah samastāsakalā jagatsu.

"All sciences are forms of Devī,

As also all women, without exception, throughout the world."

– Candi (Mārkaṇḍeya Purāṇa)

Introduction to Part II :

Hinduism as a Religion

Being a Hindu is both a way of life and a religion. The latter has been largely misunderstood and the former is rarely understood. In the second part of this book, we will attempt to understand the Hindu religion and spiritual thought process, with respect to menstruation.

The English language has become the most common language of communication across the world. A language conveys not just meanings of words, but also unconsciously influences the thought process. As a result, a language can paint a good picture or taint a culture and the associated religion, either by effectively producing the right visual imagery of that culture and religion or by superimposing the imagery of the thought process of the native speakers of the language, which might be alien to another culture and religion. The latter is what the English language did to the culture and religion of the Hindus. As a result, many fine ideas, subtle thought processes, and culturally significant practices of Hindus were distorted or reduced to fit the understanding of an English-speaking audience.

During the course of writing this book, I have, at times, made the mistake of using English words to convey ideas that belong to the Hindu thought process, with the intention of keeping it simple for the reader. But this simplification of language might result in a distortion of ideas for those who are unfamiliar with the Hindu culture and religion. I am grateful that these errors were pointed out to me by Jayant ji during his review of this book. I have tried my best to replace many such words with appropriate words from Saṃskṛtam or other Indian languages, to ensure that the thought process is not reduced or altered in the minds of the readers.

Before we step into the second part of this book, I feel that it is imperative to bring attention to certain words and how their meanings have been literally 'lost in translation'. True comprehension of a culture and/or religion becomes easier when one has an understanding of the original meaning of the words and ideas that were meant to be conveyed. In the following paragraphs are some words and ideas that are featured in the chapters that follow, which need to be understood correctly and clearly distinguished from the words and/or ideas often used to describe them in the English language. More details about these words and ideas will appear in a specific context in the chapters that follow.

1. Tantra is not about sex

Perhaps the most misunderstood science is that of Tantra. Promoted in the West as techniques of increasing the duration of sexual climax, Tantra has become synonymous with secretive and esoteric sexual rituals. This reduction in the meaning of Tantra is indicative of a collective thought process that revolves around sexuality. So, what is Tantra, and why did it originate?

In Hinduism, human existence is understood to belong to the four Yugas or epoch ages, namely the Satya Yuga, Tretā

Yuga, Dvāpara Yuga, and Kali Yuga. Each Yuga is associated with a decreasing ability of humans to attain mokṣa (spiritual liberation), which is considered as the ultimate aim of human birth. Accordingly, for each Yuga, a different type of Śāstra (sacred text) is said to be appropriate.

For the Satya Yuga, the Śāstra as Śruti (that which has been heard) containing revelation of the highest truth as propounded in the Vedas, and revealed to ṛṣis (seers) in deep states of subtle consciousness (samādhi), are prescribed. For the Tretā Yuga, the Śāstra as Smṛti (that which has been remembered) are prescribed. For the Dvāpara Yuga, the Purāṇas are prescribed, which contain deep ideas and ways to attain mokṣa explained in the form of simple stories. For the present age of Kali Yuga, what is prescribed is the Āgama Śāstra/Tantra Śāstra[1], which lays down the rules, rituals, discipline, and methods of sādhana required to experience the essence of the Vedas, taking into account the inability of the majority of people (in the Kali Yuga) to follow strict discipline or even understand the deeper meaning of the Śāstra as prescribed in the Vedas, Smṛti, or Purāṇa.

The Hindu religion, as it exists today, cannot be understood without the correct knowledge of Tantra Śāstra. Tantra Śāstra itself cannot be understood by mere intellectualization or reading of books. In a letter written to Sir John Woodroff by Pandit Shiva Chandra Vidyārnava, the author of the Tantratattva, he writes:[2]

> "At the present time, the general public is ignorant of the principles of the Tantra Śāstra. The cause of this ignorance is the fact that the Tantra Śāstra is a Sādhana Śāstra, the greater part of which becomes intelligible only by sādhana.

> For this reason, the Śāstra and their teachers prohibit their promulgation[...] Tantra Śāstra is broadly divided into three parts, namely sādhana, siddhi (that which is gained by sādhana) and philosophy (darśana).
>
> The special virtue of Tantra lies in its mode of sādhana. It is neither mere worship nor prayer. It is not lamenting or contrition or repentance before the deity. It is the sādhana which is the union of puruṣa (male principle/ consciousness) with prakṛti (female principle within the body). It is the object of Tantrik sādhana to merge the self-principle (Svarāt) into the Universal (Virāt). A man is considered a siddha in this sādhana when he is able to awaken the kuṇḍalinī and pierce the six cakras."

Kularnava Tantra says that knowledge alone can gain spiritual liberation. Knowledge in the sense of the Śāstra is actual immediate experience (sākṣātkāra). This knowledge is gained by following the methods and discipline prescribed in the form of sādhana in Tantra. Sādhana is derived from the root of the word 'sadh', which means 'to exert'. Sādhana is of many types based on the outcome that is associated with it. The rituals and practices associated with the Hindu religion such as pūjā, mantra japā, various forms of yōg, dhyāna, etc. are different types of sādhana. Religion often influences the culture of a region and vice versa. Therefore, many of the cultural practices of Hindus have their foundation in Tantra.

The reason for Tantra being notoriously associated with sex is that there are few practices where the sādhaka (one undertaking the sādhana) is taught to work with sexual energy and channelize it for a spiritual purpose. Rather than promote sexual activity, such sādhana teaches one to restrain basic sexual urges and use sexual energy for raising the kuṇḍalinī[3] as part of a spiritual process.

Tantra texts which prescribe these practices are clear with instructions of who is not eligible for such practice (for example, one who has no control over his sexual urges should not attempt such techniques). Moreover, none of these practices should be attempted without the guidance of a genuine Guru, nor should it be discussed publicly, to prevent misunderstanding and misuse. The practical application of Tantra is such that it took into consideration the workings of the human mind in the Kali Yuga. Sexual urges are the most difficult to overcome and restrain in the path of spirituality. Therefore, instead of merely prescribing moral discipline and abstinence from sex, Tantra taught methods of transforming the sexual energy for a higher spiritual purpose. The use of Tantra for mere sexual satisfaction is an indication of the extent to which humans have degenerated in the Kali Yuga. The reduction of Tantra to sexual rituals is indicative of a collective ignorance of the Śāstra.

Tantra does not ask anyone to have blind faith or follow instructions without inquiry. Instead, it teaches that if one desires to renounce anything, it should be renounced only after a thorough acquaintance with it; if one desires to embrace anything new, it should be embraced only after a searching inquiry[2] - a principle which applies to all that is written in this book.

2. Prāṇa Pratiṣṭhā is not symbolic consecration

The Oxford dictionary mentions that to consecrate something means 'to state officially in a religious ceremony that something is holy and can be used for religious purposes'. The word consecration in English is often used in association with the Christian belief to make bread and wine into the body and blood of Christ (Holy Eucharist). The process which transforms the bread and wine into the body and blood of Christ is itself largely considered as only symbolic, and consequently, even the word consecration has come to mean something that is symbolically sacred.

Prāṇa Pratiṣṭhā is often translated as 'consecration' in works describing Hindu temples and therefore assigned only symbolic meaning, by those who are only familiar with the popular Western notion of consecration. Whereas, Āgama Śāstra describes the technique of prāṇa pratiṣṭhā as a process that infuses prāṇa (life force) into a specific object or space. In other words, prāṇa pratiṣṭhā enables manifestation of the Devatā Śakti in a form that humans can experience, and not just symbolically or mentally associate with. It is the technique of prāṇa pratiṣṭhā that transforms a stone sculpture into a mūrti/ vigraha as a living presence of the deity invoked. This does not mean that a spiritual experience is only possible in a temple or that God (as is often understood) is present only in a temple. In Hinduism, the correct word for God is Brahman, which refers to the ultimate source of the entire cosmos. Brahman is understood as Nirguṇa, meaning that without form (or gender).

As we entered Kali Yuga, Tantra Śāstra understood that majority of us cannot relate to the abstract concept of Brahman, without concrete form. And therefore, Tantra introduced Hindu temples which enable the manifestation of Brahman in the Saguṇa (with form) aspect with various attributes, each named as a particular Deva (masculine form of a deity) or Devī (feminine form of a deity). The science and technique of prāṇa pratiṣṭhā make this manifestation possible.

3. Caitanyam is not energy

Speakers of the English language use and abuse the word 'energy' whenever something is difficult to explain, owing to a lack of perception by the ordinary senses. Therefore, the presence in a Hindu temple is often loosely termed as energy. The term used in many Indian languages to indicate the nature of that which is invoked by the process of prāṇa pratiṣṭhā is known as caitanya or caitanyam. The best way to understand the nature of a particular Hindu temple is by experiencing the caitanyam in that temple—sometimes perceived at once by those who have tuned themselves to recognize subtle experiences, and at other times, by the after-effect of visiting that particular temple.

Not all temples are alike, even if the deity is in the same form. This has to do with the nature of the caitanyam, which is the result of the saṅkalpa (intention) put into the process of prāṇa pratiṣṭhā. This is why the original rules prescribed for rituals in a temple are generally not tampered with, since only the person who undertook the prāṇa pratiṣṭhā will know what exactly he put in there and how to maintain the caitanyam in that temple. Even to change methods of offering (for example, replacing animal sacrifices with vegetables such as pumpkin) requires a qualified practitioner who is an authority on Āgama/ Tantra Śāstra and is capable of understanding the nature of the caitanyam and saṅkalpa, in order to alter the process without interfering with it.

4. Upāsana is not worship

Worship is defined as 'to honor or show reverence for a divine being or supernatural power', according to Merriam-Webster dictionary. This definition brings to mind a relationship between two distinct entities—the worshipper and the worshipped—which are considered as separate, with the worshipper never daring to consider himself/herself as one with the worshipped.

Upāsana, on the other hand, refers to the process which brings the devotee closer to the Devata and eventually results in the devotee experiencing oneness with the Devata. It is said that regular Upāsana of one's Iṣṭa Devata (preferred form of the deity chosen by the devotee) results in the Upāsak (one doing the Upāsana) resembling the Iṣṭa Devata in form, manner, and likeness.

An example of the closeness of the relationship with his Iṣṭa Devata is beautifully expressed in ancient poems and songs where the composer pretends to be angry with or playfully teases his Iṣṭa Devata, out of love. The works of 17th century Telugu composer Bhadrachala Ramadasu, wherein he asks Bhagvan Ram 'why have your words become as rare as gold?' (paluke bangaramayena?), is a popular example of such closeness. Similarly, the celebrated Kannada poet Purandaradasa takes liberty with teasing Devī Lakṣmī as 'Venkataramanana binkada rani', meaning 'the haughty queen of Venkataramana', in the famous composition 'Bhāgyada Lakṣmī bāramma'. Followers of Hinduism as a religion often express fondness for the Devata, which is usually reserved for someone very close to him/her, through Upāsana which includes bathing, adoring with flowers and fragrance, feeding, and even singing a lullaby for the invoked Devata. For an Upāsak, the object of their Upāsana, the Iṣṭa Devata, is with them at all times.

At times, the word 'worship' is used to indicate pūjā. In the context of a Hindu temple, pūjā refers to the rituals that help in maintaining the caitanyam in the temple. The person officiating the pūjā in a Hindu temple is called a pūjāri, pandit, arcaka, melśānti, or tantrī based on the language.

5. Śakti is not a Goddess

English works on Hindu deities use the word 'Goddess' to refer to the feminine form of a deity and 'God' to refer to the masculine form. The Merriam-Webster dictionary defines the word 'Goddess' as 'a female God', indicating that God is male and the Goddess is a form of, and therefore lower in the hierarchy to, a male God. This is a clear influence of a thought process that is inherently patriarchal, so much so that even a Goddess has to be defined under the shadow of a male God.

In the Hindu religion, rather than male and female demarcations, there is the understanding of two opposite principles, puruṣa and prakṛti. Puruṣa refers to the changeless aspect of Brahman, while prakṛti refers to the ever-changing quality of Brahman waiting to manifest itself. Puruṣa is the static consciousness that cannot create on its own, while prakṛti is the dynamic creative power that cannot become conscious on its own. Therefore, according to the Sāṃkhya Darśana, it is the coming together of puruṣa and prakṛti that results in creation. In the process of simplifying this idea, puruṣa came to be referred to as the masculine principle and prakṛti as the feminine principle. Further concretization of these concepts resulted in the names Śiva and Śakti, with Śakti referring to the creative aspect of Śiva. The many names of Śakti include Mahāmaya, Viśnumāya, Parāśakti, and so on. The many forms of Śakti are who we refer to as Devī.

Creation is said to be made possible because of the will (icchā) of Brahman to manifest in many forms. This icchā is Śakti. Śakti is not separate from, nor can Śakti be separated from, Brahman. The universe is simply an opening out (unmeṣa) or expansion (prasāra) of Brahman as Śakti. Śakti is the first cause; the cause of all causes. Śakti is what manifests, sustains, and transforms the universe as the one unifying force of existence. Śakti is not exclusive to a religion, class, or cult and is universal.

The Kubjikā Tantra says: "Whosoever has seen the feet of woman let him worship them as those of his guru" (Strinām pādatalam driṣtvāguruvadbhāvayet sadā). While male and female are both Her aspects, yet Śakti is, in a sense, said to be more revealed in the female than in the male form. And so, the Muṇḍamāla Tantra says: "Wherever there is a Śaktī (female), there I am." On account of this greater manifestation, women are called Śakti.[4]

The concept of the creator as a Divine Mother existed since time immemorial but has been lost to most cultures across the world. Woodroffe, in his book Shakti and Shakta, reminds us of this universality, when he writes:

> "For, when we throw our minds back upon the history of this worship we see stretching away into the remote and fading past the figure of the Mighty Mother of Nature, most ancient among the ancients; the Ādya Śakti, the dusk divinity, many breasted crowned with towers whose veil

is never lifted, Isis, "the one who is all that has been, is, and will be", Kāli, Hathor, Cybele, the Cowmother Goddess Ida, Tripurasundari, the Ionic Mother, Tef the spouse of Shu by whom He effects the birth of all things, Aphrodite, Astrate in whose groves the Baalim were set, Babylonian Mylitta, Buddhist Tārā, the Mexican Ish, Hellenic Osia, the consecrated, the free and pure, African Salambo, who like Pārvati roamed the mountains, Roman Juno, Egyptian Bast the flaming Mistress of Life, of Thought, of Love, whose festival was celebrated with wanton joy, the Assyrian Mother Succoth Benoth, Northern Freia, Mūlāprakrti, Semele, Māyā, Ishtar, Saitic Neith Mother of the Gods, eternal deepest ground of all things, kuṇḍali, Guhyamahābhairavi and all the rest."

The need of the hour is for women across the world to dig deeper and unearth their own ancestral memory and ways of acknowledging the Divine as Feminine, and not just borrow Hindu concepts of Śakti or Devī and reduce it to 'a female God'.

Menstruation in the Hindu religion

On the face of it, it may seem to many that the treatment of menstruating women in India is contradictory. On the one hand, India has the rare (perhaps, only) temples dedicated to menstruating Devīs[5], where Her menstruation is a cause for community celebration, while on the other hand, menstruating women are told not to enter a temple until their period is over. How do we explain this seeming contradiction?

Mīmāmsā darśana, which prescribes the methodology to arrive at the correct meaning of the Vedas, speaks of contradiction as an error in understanding the Vedas.

Mīmāmsā says that if we come across ideas or rules that seem contradictory or incongruent with what is otherwise stated, it means that there is a gap in our understanding. Since all forms of Hindu religious practices are but different expressions of the teaching in the Vedas, the rules pertaining to temple visits for women must also not be contradictory to the idea of women as a manifestation of Śakti. In the second part of this book, we will try and resolve this seeming contradiction, with the help of Tantra Śāstra.

Of all the menstrual regulations that young girls and women have sought answers for, the foremost are those pertaining to visiting Hindu temples at the time of menstruation. This is the most difficult question to come to terms with. The question "Am I so impure during menstruation that even the Devatās do not want to see me?" asked innocently by young girls would compel anyone to take up a deeper study on the subject. It was this question that led me on a mission of sorts, to get to the root of the answer.

I find it illogical to accept that our ancestors were such misogynists that they deviously planned restrictions on menstruating women, just to suppress them. The special place for women in the Hindu religion and the reverence of the Divine Feminine, which is alive in India even when most of the world has buried it, makes one think twice about what the missing link might be. It took me years of traveling to different parts of India, of interacting with learned men and women, of seeking guidance from spiritual masters, of learning the science behind Hindu temples, and most significantly, of experiencing the caitanyam in Hindu temples, to arrive at the answers. And yet, I know I have only touched the tip of a very large iceberg.

What I am about to share in the following pages is much more than a theory of scientific knowledge about religion or spirituality. What I am about to share is experience—what a woman's body can experience and how it can lead the way for a deeper understanding of subtler realms.

It is indeed a wonder that a subject like menstruation, when dug deeper, can take one so far.

References for Introduction to Part II

1. While Āgama refers to a tradition, Tantra is a technique. But both share the same ideology.
2. Woodroffe, Sir John: Shakti and Shakta, 1925
3. Kuṇḍalinī is a term used to refer to a fundamental life force that lies dormant in the lowest cakra called mūlādhāra. The rising of the kuṇḍalinī is accomplished by certain sādhana, causing it to pierce through the six cakras and reach the sahasrāra or the seat of consciousness. When this happens, the spiritual aspirant is said to be able to experience oneness with the cosmos, or in other words, experience self-realization.
4. Woodroffe: Hymns to the Goddess, 1913
5. Bhagavathi Devī temple in Chengannur, Kerala and Kāmakhya Devī temple in Guwahati, Assam

CHAPTER 8

HOW DO HINDU TEMPLES IMPACT MENSTRUATION?

To understand Hindu temples and the impact that they have on the human physiology, we need to set aside conditioned ideas of religion and belief systems. The most essential aspect required to understand an unfamiliar subject is an open mind.

I have, sometimes, been asked the question "Why Hindu temples? Why not study about churches or mosques or gurudwaras?" While there is a chapter in this book that explores the menstrual regulations in Christianity, Islam, and the absence of such regulations in the Sikh religion, it is important to state that my understanding of other religions was greatly enhanced by understanding the Hindu religion.

The reason I chose Hindu temples as a subject of study is not just because it is the religion of the majority population in India, but also because it is the mother of all ancient religions and encompasses all the faiths, doctrines, and theories of other religions. It is this understanding of all paths as being valid means that makes the Hindu accept all faiths and doctrines, and not merely 'tolerate' other religions.

The seed

While attempting to find answers to the difficult question of why women are restricted from entering Hindu temples during menstruation, Jayant ji directed me to the Devīpuram temple in Andhra Pradesh. This temple has been constructed as a three-dimensional representation of the sacred Śrī Cakra[1] itself. I was fascinated to learn that this temple had women pūjāri, and certain portions of the temple, such as the Kāmākhya pīṭha, were welcome to menstruating women as well. I visited Devīpuram sometime in early 2015, in search of answers. After all, who better to learn from than one who has experienced the Divine Feminine?

It was my meeting with Guruji, Pūjya Śrī Amritānanda Nātha Saraswathi, a top nuclear physicist turned exponent of the sacred Śrī Vidyā, that completely turned my perspective on the rhetoric of women being impure during menstruation. At that time, I had written to several prominent spiritual masters, seeking their interview. The only response I got was from Guruji. As I now look back, I realize that it was the only response I needed.

In response to my question regarding regulations on menstruating women from entering temples, this was his answer:

> "What is pure, we do not touch. And what we do not touch, we call it a taboo. She (a menstruating woman) was so pure, that she was worshipped as a Goddess. The reason for not having a woman go into a temple is precisely this. She is a living Goddess at that time. The energy of the God or Goddess which is there in the mūrti will move over to

her, and that becomes lifeless, while this (the menstruating woman) is life. So, that's why they were prevented from entering the temple. So, it is exactly the opposite of what we think."

Guruji's fascinating response made me look at the entire subject in a whole new light, turning it over and over in my mind, until many more unanswered questions surfaced. Every time I found one answer, it led to a series of more questions. I never could meet Guruji again, and he left his physical body later that same year. My brief interaction with him and a book on his work, Gifts from the Goddess,[2] continue to help me find answers to new questions, every time I read it.

To be or not to be, a woman or a Devī?

Guruji's words pointed to positive reasoning for regulations on menstruating women and answered the question of why a menstruating woman's presence in a temple is considered to be an act of displeasing and disrespecting the deity. When temple authorities learn of a disturbance in the caitanyam,[3] they have to undertake elaborate rituals to restore the caitanyam of the mūrti and of the place. However, this is not the only reason why women are discouraged from visiting temples during menstruation. The other important reason is the answer to the question 'how would entering the temple impact a menstruating woman?'

Before I begin the explanation to this, we need to understand that for all such questions, there are different levels of understanding, based on each of our inclination to dig deeper. Some of us might find the simple answer of women needing rest during menstruation to be sufficient, and that is fine. Others may feel the need to go deeper and learn about the science behind it, and that is fine too. Unless the answers are contradictory, it is safe to assume that they are all correct; the difference is only in the depth of understanding.

Prāṇa pratiṣṭhā

What sets apart a Hindu temple from other places of worship is that the entire building of a temple has a living presence. Every pillar, every stone, every step, every section is imbibed with a certain power by virtue of the process called prāṇa pratiṣṭhā. Sometimes, the word 'consecration' is used to assign an English term for prāṇa pratiṣṭhā, but it should be understood that in the context of the Hindu religion, prāṇa pratiṣṭhā goes beyond symbolism of something sacred and refers to a technique of invoking the presence of the deity into a physical location.

The frequently used Saṃskṛtam term for consecration is pratiṣṭhā, which is uttered in the ritual Om prati-tiṣṭha parameśvara, meaning 'O Parameśvara, abide here'.[4] When prāṇa pratiṣṭhā is done effectively, it has an influence on the devotee, not just spiritually, but also physiologically.

The nature of the caitanyam in a temple determines the effect it has on humans. A devotee might have visited hundred or more Devī temples, but each one could have a different impact on the devotee, based on the nature of the caitanyam and saṅkalpam that is imbibed in the mūrti and in the space. While this subject is not easy to theorize, it is possible to know it through a direct experience of such spaces. This aspect of experiencing the caitanyam in a temple is described in the subsequent chapters of this book.

In Hindu temples, the mūrti is never made for the purpose of the temple, but rather that the temple is constructed and prepared as an outward manifestation of the deity whose presence has been invoked into the mūrti. The temple that is built is likened to the body and the deity installed in it to the soul. Thus, providing a body for the soul is the purpose of constructing the temple. In the Āgama and Śilpa Śāstra texts, the parts of the temple are known by the names of the limbs of the human body. For example, pāda (feet), ūru (thigh), gala (throat), nāsikā (nose), karṇa (ear), mukha (mouth), śira (head), kaṭī (waist), bhuja (hand), etc. The rituals involved in the construction of the temple are therefore planned to provide an adequate body for the deity.

Several ancient Hindu temples in South India are constructed based on the site plan called vāstu puruṣa maṇḍala; it personifies a human-like form called vāstu puruṣa, the site deity, whose entire body (drawn facing downwards) covers the site plan, which usually has 64 or 81 square cells. The mid-most square of four cells is regarded as the heart of the vāstu puruṣa and is the location of the Brahma (brahma-sthāna). The area of the sanctum is the brahma-sthāna of the shrine complex.

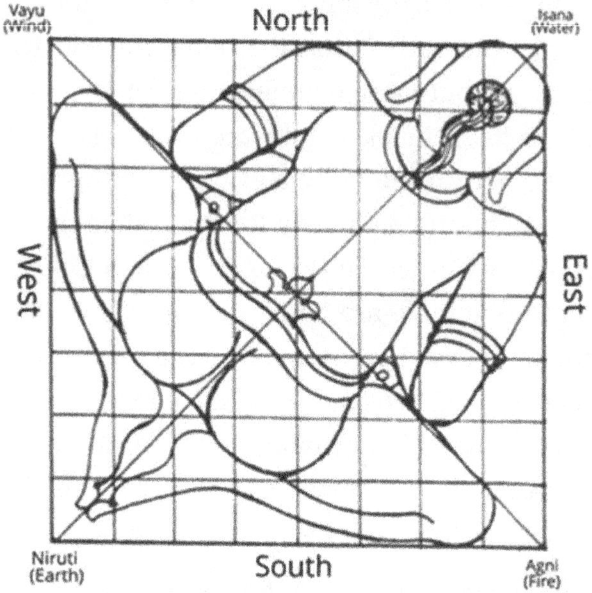

Figure 5: Vastu Purusha Mandala
(Image Source: By Verena Rapp de Eston - Own work, CC BY-SA 4.0, httpscommons.wikimedia.orgwindex.phpcurid=43730422)

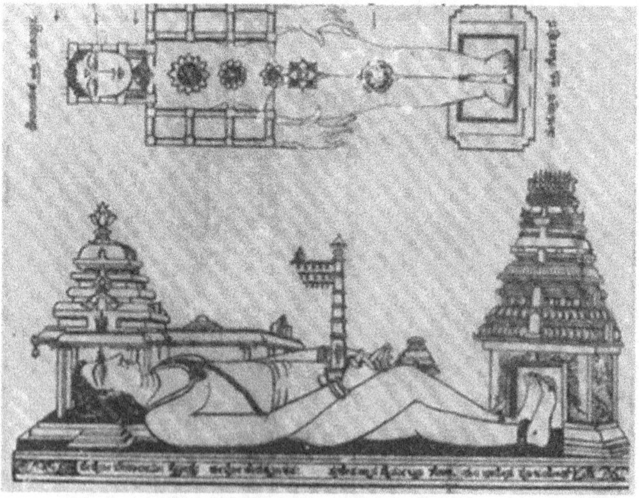

Figure 6: Manushya Devalaya,
(Source: Rao, S.K.Ramachandra. The Agama Encyclopedia, 2005)

S. K. Ramachandra Rao's book[5] explains how the ancient texts compare the temple to the likeness of a human form: "As a temple is laid out, it is said to picture a man (the vāstu puruṣa) lying down. His feet connote the entrance tower, his genital organ the flag-staff (dhvaja-stambha), his belly the assembly hall (ranga maṇḍapa), his heart the porch (antarāla), his head the sanctum and the brow-meet (space between eyebrows) the seat of the icon."

Hindu temples are classified based on several aspects such as architectural plan shapes, number of storeys, decorations, space utilization, construction materials used, location, type and pose of the mūrti, region in India, etc. When it comes to the process and rituals of maintaining the caitanyam, we gain insights from the classification of temples into five types by texts like Padma-purāṇa and Parameśvara Saṃhita, as follows:

a. Svayam-Vyakta – where the image is a self-manifestation
b. Daivika – created by celestial beings in ancient times in very pure places or mountain tops
c. Ārṣa – built by ancient sages in forests, by the power of their penance
d. Paurānas – those acclaimed in the Purānas
e. Mānuṣa – built by humans in recent times

The texts insist that when it is a self-manifest image or those installed by ancient sages, no prāṇa pratiṣṭhā is needed. If the mūrti is an ancient one but has been without worship for a length of time, prāṇa pratiṣṭhā may be done, but without the sequence of immersion in water, milk, grains, etc. to avoid removing it from the spot where prāṇa pratiṣṭhā was done in the past. If it is removed, it is said to spell ruin for the country.

Cakras

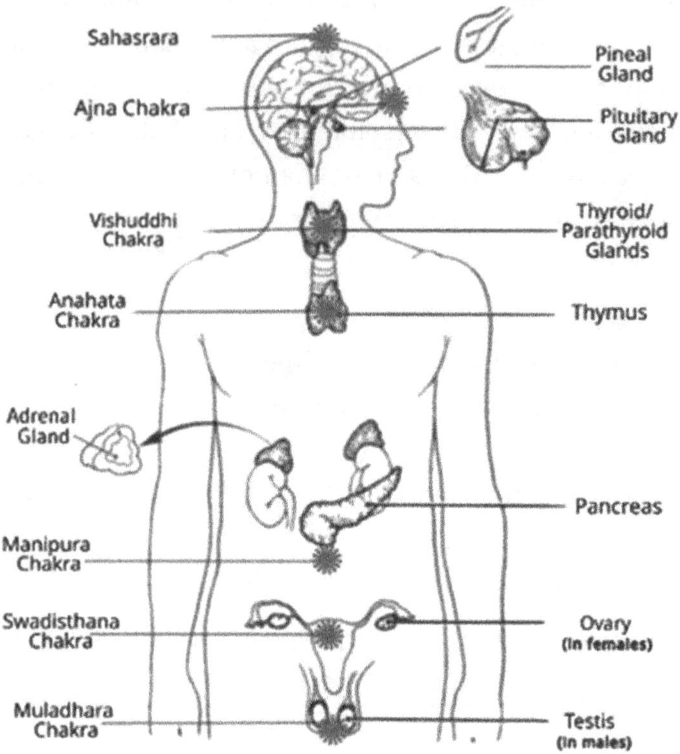

Figure 7: Cakras and endocrine glands

How does a Hindu temple impact a human being? The answer to this lies in the science of cakras. I have explained cakras with relation to Hindu temples in my book Women and Sabarimala[6], which can be referred to for more information. A brief description of the six cakras is given in the Notes section of this book, titled 'Ṣat Cakras: The Six Cakras'. Here, an overview is presented.

Just as we recognize nerves and plexus points in the sthūla śarīra (gross anatomy), Indian sciences understood that there are nāḍīs and cakras in the sūkṣma śarīra (subtle anatomy).

Cakras are energy junctions in the sūkṣma śarīra where several nāḍīs (subtle energy channels) meet and branch out, carrying the vital life-force, prāṇa, to various parts of the body. Although there are a few hundred cakras, we largely focus on six cakras arranged along the spinal column. These six cakras are presented in the diagram below. There is also a seventh Sahasrāra cakra, which some do not categorize as a cakra and instead refer to as the seat of pure consciousness.

Each cakra in turn influences specific doṣas in its region of operation as well as endocrine glands and their corresponding organs (see diagram). For the purpose of understanding menstruation, it is important to note that the two lowest cakras, viz., mūlādhāra and svadhiṣṭhāna, correspond to the excretory and reproductive system. When these two cakras are not sufficiently energized, the functions associated with the reproductive system begin to suffer.

Several temples, especially those dedicated to a Devī associated with fertility, have the prāṇa pratiṣṭhā done in such a way that the caitanyam in such spaces energize the mūlādhāra and svadhiṣṭhāna cakras and associated nāḍīs, thereby infusing the reproductive organs with prāṇa and helping women with menstrual and reproductive disorders experience healing.

To summarize, temples affect one or more cakras based on the nature of the caitanyam. The cakras in turn affect endocrine glands, associated organs, and also doṣas, thereby influencing human physiology.

Subtypes of doṣas

To understand how temples impact doṣas, we need to delve deeper into the understanding of subtypes of doṣas, especially those of the vāta doṣa. A basic introduction to vāta doṣa and its role in menstruation has been covered in the previous section of the book. As mentioned earlier, vāta doṣa is dominant during menstruation, as it aids the movement of menstrual blood down and out of the body. Vāta doṣa has five subtypes, each facilitating specific functions in different parts of the body.

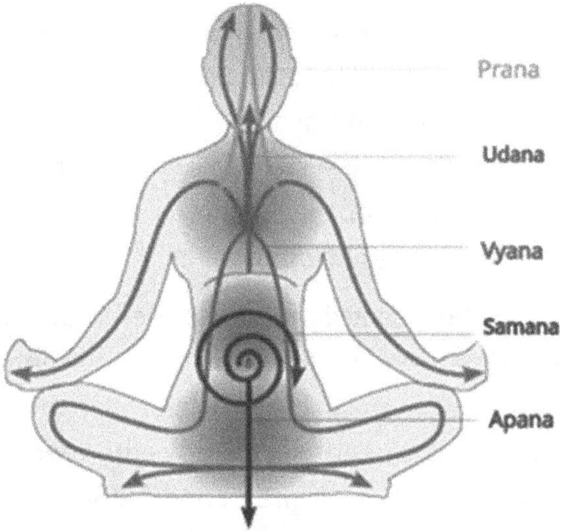

Figure 8: Five types of vāta doṣa

1. **Prāṇa** – Prāṇa vāyu is responsible for the downward and inward movement of breath or, in other words, inhalation. It is also responsible for pushing food into the stomach cavity, through the act of swallowing. Prāṇa vāyu dominates the region of the head but also moves to other regions to facilitate certain processes in those regions as well. Often, the words breath and prāṇa

are used interchangeably. It is important to note that breath is one of the functions of prāṇa, but prāṇa itself is not limited to breath. The term prāṇa is also used to represent the vital life force that is responsible for life itself. Prāṇa vāyu, which is the subtype of vāta doṣa, is one of the aspects of the life-force Prāṇa and should be understood in the context mentioned.

2. **Udāna** – Udāna vāyu is responsible for the upward movement of breath, or exhalation, and is dominant in the throat and chest region. It controls the functions in the throat and also controls speech. All upward and outward movements such as vomiting and burping occur due to the udāna vāyu. Many of us would have been advised to avoid talking while eating. The reason is that speech is controlled by the upward moving udāna, while the downward moving prāṇa is responsible for forcing the food down. If these two opposite forces are activated simultaneously, the chances of choking are high.

3. **Vyāna** – Vyāna vāyu is the all-pervading vāyu which moves in all directions within the body. It controls the functions of the heart and circulatory system. Diseases that affect the entire body, such as fever, are said to be due to a deranged vyāna vāyu.

4. **Samāna** – Samāna vāyu is the vāta subtype which moves in the stomach region. It is this vāyu which is responsible for the process of digestion and for disintegrating the essence of food from refuse or excreted matter. When samāna vāyu is not functioning properly, digestive issues like dysentery will occur. Unknown to many Indians, the routine gesture of moving the hand in a circular

clockwise manner over the stomach soon after a meal is an unconscious act of triggering of the samāna vāyu to aid digestion.

5. **Apāna** – Apāna vāyu is the most significant vāta subtype for understanding menstruation, reproduction, and associated disorders. Apāna is the downward moving force which controls the downward and outward functions of urination, defecation, menstruation, release of semen (in men), and childbirth. It acts in the lower region of the intestine. If the downward movement of apāna vāyu is obstructed in any way or is forced to change its direction, women will experience difficulty in menstruation.

   A change in the direction of apāna vāyu will also cause difficulty during childbirth since the pushing out of the fetus is a function of the downward moving apāna. To facilitate easy delivery and to trigger apāna vāyu, ancient Indian women and women in some tribes even today prefer the squatting positing for birthing. Ancient sculptures of women and Devī in the delivery position, such as that of Lajja Gowri,[7] show them in the squatting position.

Impact of Hindu temples on physiology

Ancient Hindu temples and recitation of certain mantras act on specific cakras to cause a specific impact on the devotee. In order to simplify the understanding, we can broadly classify temples into those that facilitate the aspect of worldly life (bhukti) predominantly, and those that facilitate the pursuit of the spiritual path (mukti) predominantly. This does not mean that a temple meant for mukti will not help the devotee with aspects of bhukti or vice versa. For example, the Kāmākhya temple in Assam facilitates both bhukti and mukti. Many temples, such as Śiva temples, though meant for mukti, will also have an adjoining shrine of Devī to balance the effect. Based on the purpose of the temple, the type of prāṇa pratiṣṭhā and nature of the caitanyam will be different, the temple's influence on apāna vāyu will be different, and accordingly, it will have an impact on women's menstrual cycles. Let us look at the two categories of temples and their impact on women.

Temples for bhukti

Temples that enable bhukti (worldly life) act on the physical body and resolve problems related to health and well-being. Such temples usually energize the lower cakras influencing apāna vāyu and samāna vāyu in its region of operation and rectify any changes in its movement. These temples resolve problems related to procreation, health, and well-being, as they energize the lower cakras of mūlādhāra, svadhiṣṭhāna, and maṇipūra, influencing the endocrine glands such as ovaries/testes, adrenal gland, and pancreas.

Temples focusing on prosperity and well-being have not one devathā (deity) but several along with their consorts, representing the feminine power, Śakti. Several temples dedicated to the grāma devathā (village deity) work on the mūlādhāra cakra and help devotees overcome basic survival difficulties. Temples dedicated to a fertility Devī, typically visited on Tuesdays and Fridays, act on the svadhiṣṭhāna cakra and help devotees with problems pertaining to reproductive health. Temples that are famous for healing specific ailments, such as the Venni Karumbeshwarar Temple (Tamil Nadu), known to cure diabetes, act on the maṇipūra cakra and resolve problems pertaining to the adrenal gland and pancreas. Similarly, the Achankovil Dharma Sastha temple in Kerala, which acts on the svadhiṣṭhāna cakra, is known for curing snake and other venomous insect bites. These are only a few examples of temples that help devotees in day-to-day life and well-being.

If menstruating women visited such temples which work on the lower cakras, it could further trigger the apāna vāyu at a time when it is already in action. Menstruation causes the apāna vāyu to be active throughout the duration of the menstrual flow. At such a time, visiting temples that act on the apāna vāyu by energizing the svadhiṣṭhāna and mūlādhāra cakra could result in heavy bleeding or other menstrual disturbances.

Similar to the regulation on menstruating women from entering Hindu temples, there are general rules for all devotees pertaining to the appropriate time and method of visiting temples. The general practice followed for temple visits is to go on an empty stomach, early in the morning, after having emptied the bowels and after having a bath. For someone who just had a meal and visited a temple soon after, the action of the samāna vāyu, which would be working to digest the food consumed, will be impacted, causing digestive upsets. Not only have I experienced this during my post-lunch visit to the Aryankavu Dharma Sastha temple in Kollam (Kerala) and again in the Sugreeswarar temple in Tiruppur (Tamil Nadu), but I have heard similar experiences from others who visited a temple soon after a meal. Similarly, those who frequently undertake mantra japa or pūjā are often recommended a lighter diet or are required to fast, so that the effects of upward movement of prāṇa through such activities will have minimal impact on the digestive movement of samāna vāyu. Thus, we see that the rules and regulations pertaining to temple visits have a valid reason and an impact on the human system.

Temples for mukti

The other category of temples is those that facilitate mukti or mokṣa (spiritual liberation) as a predominant aspect. Such temples help the devotee develop vairāgya (detachment) toward worldly pursuits and propel them in the path of spirituality. These temples energize the higher cakras. When the higher cakras are triggered, it causes the apāna vāyu, if active, to change its normal downward course and turn upward.

The temple of Swamy Ayyappa at Sabarimala and other temples known as mokṣa dham (place for attaining spiritual liberation) fall in this category and are generally not advised for women in the reproductive age. In such temples, even if women are not menstruating at the time of the visit but are of the menstrual age, they are usually restricted from entering. While temples like Sabarimala have written instructions asking women between the ages of 10 to 50 years to refrain from entering, most other temples assume that devotees are aware of this rule and might not have it explicitly mentioned. In India, most women traditionally visit mokṣa dhams and take to the spiritual path only after menopause, when they have naturally completed worldly responsibilities. But why is it not recommended for women in the reproductive age to visit a mokṣa dham?

The simplest way to understand this is to realize that the process of bhukti and mukti do not go hand in hand. The body of a woman, in her reproductive years, is inclined toward the procreative process and creation of life. Whereas, the spiritual process of mukti is inclined toward the dissolution of life to eventually end the cycle of birth and re-birth. These two opposing acts of creation and dissolution cause conflict in the physical body of a woman in her reproductive years. The example of Sabarimala shrine as covered in my earlier book Women and Sabarimala is a good start to understand how mokṣa dhams impact women of reproductive age, even though they are not menstruating at the time of their visit. A similar explanation is offered in the context of the Gayatri Mantra in Chapter 10 of this book, titled 'Mantras and Their Effect on Menstrual Cycles'.

When women visit mokṣa dhams during menstruation, the pull of apāna in the opposite direction (upward) would most likely cause a perceptible pain in the lower abdomen. If continued over a period of time, such temples can cause irreparable damage by changing the direction of apāna vāyu or blocking it. This could be one of the reasons for the painful menstrual disorder called endometriosis. Modern medicine does not know the cause for endometriosis, but one of the theories suggest what is called 'retrograde menstruation', which means the menstrual blood reverses its flow and deposits itself in the fallopian tube, uterus, and sometimes even higher. This is very likely to be a case of apāna reversal, which is extremely difficult to treat.

Reversal of apāna vāyu can be caused due to other reasons as well. Any activity which causes a reversal of apāna vāyu during menstruation could cause endometriosis. For example, inverted yōga postures, gymnastics requiring inverted jumps, or even going against gravity by excessive air travel during menstruation. If these activities are undertaken month after month during menstruation, it would cause apāna vāyu to eventually change direction, thereby reversing menstrual flow or blocking it altogether.

Is there evidence?

It is likely that some of you may find the above information hard to accept. After all, where is the evidence that visiting ancient Hindu temples during menstruation can cause problems? Or for that matter, where is the evidence of the positive health impact that temples have on devotees?

Over the years, I have realized that when people ask for 'evidence', they have in mind a particular idea of what they assume evidence means. It is rarely the same. For some, evidence means that the idea/theory proposed has been mentioned in an ancient sacred text and hence is accepted as valid. For some, it has to be validated by a person(s) who they consider as a subject-matter expert or has a particular qualification. For others, evidence means research undertaken as per the framework of modern science with control groups, clinical trials, peer-reviewed, and published in what they consider as legitimate science journals.

And for a few, evidence simply means being able to have a first-hand experience of what is theorized. For one who has experienced the positive impact of these temples, like hundreds of devotees, no other evidence is needed. For one who is unwilling to make the effort through sādhana to have a positive experience, or ignores their experiences, no evidence will suffice.

Experience of women

There are many instances of devotees having experienced a positive change in their health, especially menstrual and reproductive health, after visiting certain temples. One only needs to meet and interact with the regular visitors to such temples to gather the evidence they need.

The more difficult experience to document is that of how some temples have negatively impacted women's menstrual health. When I share this information with women during my workshops or through my write-ups, women in turn share with me their personal experiences. Their experiences along with my own are what have helped me understand the scientific basis of the phenomena associated with temples. Here are a few experiences shared by some of the women of what happened when they broke the traditional regulations pertaining to visiting Hindu temples during menstruation. Their names have not been mentioned to protect their identity.

> "I wanted to share an experience I had some years ago. There were half a dozen of my friends at a meditation teacher's house for satsang and pūjā. The husband and wife explained that for those of us menstruating, we would be more comfortable sitting at the back of the room. They then offered us some more explanation, "the energy during menstruation goes downwards into the earth, (at the pūjā table, offerings, altar), the energy is going upwards. This can bring discomfort in the body.
>
> Well I was overtaken by the end of the chanting to pay my respects and bow down to the pūjā table. I didn't take a flower as offered by the teacher, as I thought that was part of what I shouldn't be doing. I deeply wanted to offer myself instead. Then I moved back to my spot on the floor, and within a few minutes experienced sensations like I never had before or since in my head and body, like I was being

pulled or twisted from both above and below! My good friend was supportive and told me it would end soon. And it did, I felt okay again after 5 minutes.

I am pleased to have had this experience and to be able to share it. Particularly when people criticize mosques with separate areas for women praying. I can tell my story and say that it is a purely practical and ancient approach.

I have come to find ways to honour Earth and Soil and Dream and Myth and Body and Movement and Wildness during menstruation now."

– Received by email in 2015

"I am a Saraswat Brahmin from Kashmir and I am a person who does not believe in blind customs or customs that involves a discrimination against anyone. So this is about the time I got married in 2001 and moved to Chennai with my husband. My father in law was visiting us in 2002 and we were taking him to the temples of the south tour. While in Chennai city, we went to a temple (Kapaleshwar temple in Mylapore). I was in my safe zone of menstrual cycle and nowhere close to my bleeding dates. In my family, I was not stopped from any Pūjā during my bleeding days. So, a temple visit wouldn't have changed even if I was. And I am one who thankfully has pretty smooth bleeding days. Not too much blood loss and pain.

So, when we enter the temple I start feeling weird. My head started reeling under some pressure. I ignored it and started walking towards the place where the deity was placed. Before I could reach there, I felt a sudden blackout and the need to sit down. While I excused myself and found a stone to just sit, I realized that I had suddenly started bleeding heavily and I suffered a massive blackout. I remember rushing out of the temple somehow and sitting outside for a while till I regained a part of myself. Being a person who puts science first in everything I just dismissed it as a regular instance of a bad cycle.

Now when I am more aware of the deity and their powers around, I am doubly sure that I wasn't supposed to be in that temple that day. The deity did not want me there and I was an unwanted guest. I respect the deity since it is his personal space and have since then started being more mindful of any religious places I go to. If they don't want you there, you shouldn't be. Simple."

– Received by email in 2019

"A few years ago, my family and I had been to the Amarnath yatra (a famous mokṣa dham). My period date was around the corner, but it never came. In fact, after visiting Amarnath, it took three months for my period to return! I never realized until now that it might have been owing to the temple visit."

– Shared during a discussion on the book Women & Sabarimala, 2019

"In our village, there is a famous temple of Kumaraswamy, which is about 1000 years old. Women are traditionally restricted from visiting the Kumaraswamy shrine, although they are allowed in the Parvati and Śiva shrines adjacent to the Kumaraswamy temple. In 1996, the government lifted the ban on women's entry, but many women from the village still hesitate to visit. Being an educated woman and a teacher, I always felt that this restriction is not correct and that women have equal rights to visit this temple. So, even though I'm well in my reproductive age, I decided to visit this temple. Strangely, that month, when my period came, I experienced heavy bleeding and was very tired. This was unusual. Now, after this workshop, I am able to understand why it happened."

– Shared during a workshop in Sandur village,
Bellary district, Karnataka, 2019

While the above women were able to immediately experience the effects of being in a Hindu temple, it is not so obvious for others. For some women, it takes years for the accumulated impact of continuously breaking menstrual regulations to manifest itself physically. They generally do not notice it until something major happens which cannot be ignored. And when it does, it can be painful and difficult to heal, as shared by the women in the paragraphs below.

"I grew up with a negative attitude towards menstruation.

More than the physical discomfort what hurt me was the isolation from pūjā on grounds of impurity. As I understood this was unfair as women were paying a price for a natural occurrence over which they had no control. I had no problem with God. My problem was with a practice for which no satisfactory explanation was given. I could have turned atheist like many women and girls I knew, to protest against the concept of menstrual impurity. But as I said, as a teenager I understood that rituals were socially designed and that they were purposely designed to disempower women. As I result, I decided to not follow the practice.

I began to perform all rituals like lighting lamps, reading the scriptures and visiting temples irrespective of my menstrual calendar. It made me feel powerful. It went on like this till I got menopausal. I suffered from extremely heavy bleeding and weakness for almost 6 years. I tried all modes of treatment including allopathy, homeopathy and Āyurved but with no relief.

Then I came across a series of literature and interacted with a few people whose intellect and integrity I respect, who advised me against participating in rituals while menstruating. I joined some healing groups where I was exposed to the understanding of physical ailments being manifestations of mental patterns. Around that time, I lost my mother too. I felt my menopausal issues were somehow linked with my anger at my mother. As I went deeper, I learnt to view her differently. She couldn't answer my questions as she didn't have any answers. I understood that though she gave up on me, she continued her own practice as she didn't view the issue of menstruation as a disability like I did. During this time, I gave up on doing my regular pūjā while in periods. My problem slowly abated. I cannot say I have understood the impact of certain energies on women's bodies but I have understood that there's a lot I do not know enough about. I have understood that there is a wisdom in the ancient practices that is not generally understood."

– Received by email in 2018

"Today's talk filled up lots of loopholes for me. I had my first period in our town Mariamman temple during the annual summer Pongal celebration. My mother is a fierce devotee of Sri Ramakrishna and has told me and my sister that the body is God-given, so is the periods. She has always said that going to temples during periods is fine, and I've always been proud of my mom's forward-thinking.

I have never had a regular period in my life, and I have never taken it seriously too. At times, I used to have cramps, but I have never made a fuss about it, as I've been taught that it is all part and parcel. I'm 38 now and only in the recent past that I knew that cycles happen regularly at a 28-day interval. But I've mostly been active and healthy, so when I consulted the doctors, they too said that the delay/ irregularity doesn't matter as I don't have any health issues/ troublesome period.

The thing that clicked with me today was when you said the regularity of the period will reflect on the women's inner stability. Recently, I myself have stopped going to temples during periods, as I started feeling something was not right. My whole life I've never had a regular period, and until now, I just did not make the connect!"

– Shared during a discussion on the book Women & Sabarimala, 2019

When a woman menstruates, her senses are at an all-time high. If these senses were turned inward, her body will no doubt tell her what it is going through. Any woman who breaks a menstrual regulation, especially of visiting ancient Hindu temples during menstruation, should be able to experience the consequences immediately, if she paid attention. And if not, it will manifest as complex disorders later on, which will be hard to ignore.

These experiences are not a recent phenomenon. The problem has been that women and the doctors they approach often fail to connect such experiences to temples. I remember when I discussed these incidents with a male gynecologist, he was initially dismissive, but as I kept narrating menstrual problems and possible reasons for it, he suddenly mentioned that he has had women patients who have come to him with complaints of menstrual disturbance after visiting certain temples. By his own admission, he had dismissed such experiences of patients because modern science has no knowledge of it. As we learn and speak of such incidents more and more, I have little doubt that more women will come forward to share and validate similar experiences of how ancient Hindu temples impact menstrual health.

Freedom to decide

In discussions pertaining to the case of the Sabarimala temple, some people have asked the question 'why not present the facts and leave it to women to choose what to do?' Or 'what if women are not keen on having children and choose to visit mokṣa dhams?'

Such questions arise from the limited understanding of menstruation as a switch that can be turned off and on, affecting women's ability to reproduce, and nothing more. When, in fact, any irregularity in women's menstrual cycles can impact their overall health and well-being. The effects could include obesity due to hormonal imbalance, severe dysmenorrhea, PCOS, and painful conditions like endometriosis. Even to pursue the spiritual path, good health is a fundamental requirement; and for women, good health is synonymous with good menstrual health. As the great poet Kalidasa beautifully put it[8]:

शरीरमाद्यं खलु धर्मसाधनम्

śarīramādyaṃ khalu dharmasādhanam

"The body is the foremost instrument for pursuing dharma."

Replacing fear with knowledge

It is very likely that, like me, you too might wonder as to how we lost the knowledge of the science behind Hindu temples and how we ended up distorting the meaning of the regulations to inculcate the fear of disrespecting the deity. When we study the Āgama Śāstra texts which prescribe the details of temple construction, prāṇa pratiṣṭhā, and rituals, we will observe that what is largely given are rules and not the reasons behind the rules. The Āgama texts are divided into four pāda or parts, viz.,

1. Jñāna or Vidyā pāda, dealing with philosophical and theoretical aspects
2. Yōg pāda, dealing with aspects of being in union with the divine
3. Kriyā pāda, dealing with rituals
4. Caryā pāda, dealing with the conduct of the person performing the rituals and other observances

The first two pādas deal with spiritual liberation (mukti). And the second two deal with prosperity in worldly life (bhukti). Today, the first two books which offered the philosophical and scientific reasoning of Hindu temples have been lost or ignored. What is available and followed today are the last two pādas, which are strictly adhered to during pūja and rituals. This partly explains why most temple pandits will not be able to explain the science behind the rules, rituals, and prāṇa pratiṣṭhā, even though they follow it to a T. However, through their experience, they will be aware of the impact of the rituals and the effect the temple has on devotees.

I do not doubt that there was a time in India when the knowledge of subtle sciences was not uncommon. But the more we distanced ourselves from such knowledge, the more necessary it became to provide superficial reasons and inculcate fear, instead of knowledge. Our elders could not risk women's reproductive health being impacted by walking into temples during menstruation. Instilling fear was the easier way to keep women safe; after all, we have a Hindu temple in just about every second or third street in every city, town, and village in India.

Replacing religious fear with religious knowledge is no doubt going to be a herculean task, but one that will have to be done if we are to prevent an unprecedented rise in menstrual and reproductive disorders in the years to come, as more and more women challenge traditional practices without an understanding of its purpose.

References for Chapter 8

1. Śrī Cakra is a sacred, complex, geometry used for connecting with the Divine Feminine in the Śrī Vidyā school of Hinduism.
2. Bowden, Michael. M. Gifts from the Goddess. 2017. 45th Parallel Press
3. Deva praśnam is a method of astrology (popular in Kerala) which is used to determine the state of the caitanyam in the temple, and the reason for it. For ex., in one of the temples, the reason for the presiding deity Ma Durga's absence and instead the presence of Ma Kāli, was given as entry into the temple by women in their period, presence of the spirit of the dead person, and so on. Source: Shyamasundara Dasa, 'Ashtamangala Deva Prashna', copyright 1996. https://shyamasundaradasa.com/, Lessons in Hindu Astrology (1997).
4. Rao, Ramachandra S.K, The Agama Encyclopedia. Volume IX. Consecrations, 2005
5. Rao, Ramachandra S.K., Agama Encyclopedia: Volume VI. Alaya and Aradhana, 2005
6. Joseph, Sinu. Women and Sabarimala: Science behind Restrictions. Notion Press, 2019
7. Lajja Gowri temple in Bijapur district of Karnataka is a Devī associated with fertility, depicted in the squatting position employed during child birthing
8. Kumārasambhavam by Mahakavi Kalidasa [5.33]

CHAPTER 9

CHENGANNUR BHAGAVATHY: THE TEMPLE THAT ALIGNS MENSTRUAL CYCLES

> "Experience is the only source of knowledge. Experience is the only teacher we have. We may talk and reason all our lives, but we shall not understand a word of truth, until we experience it ourselves."
>
> - Swami Vivekananda

The actual physical experience of women whose menstrual cycles have been impacted by Hindu temples is the easiest way in which we can really know the truth about the theory I have thus far explained. My own direct experience of how temples can shift menstrual cycles and impact overall health is an experience I chanced upon unknowingly when I visited the Śrī Mahadevar temple (also called Bhagavathy Temple) in Chengannur, Kerala, sometime in October 2014. My intention in visiting this temple was fairly straightforward—I wanted to learn about the menstrual festival, thriputh-aarattu, celebrated in this temple. Only in retrospect did I realize that this temple paved the way for a much more profound experience.

The Bhagavathy Temple

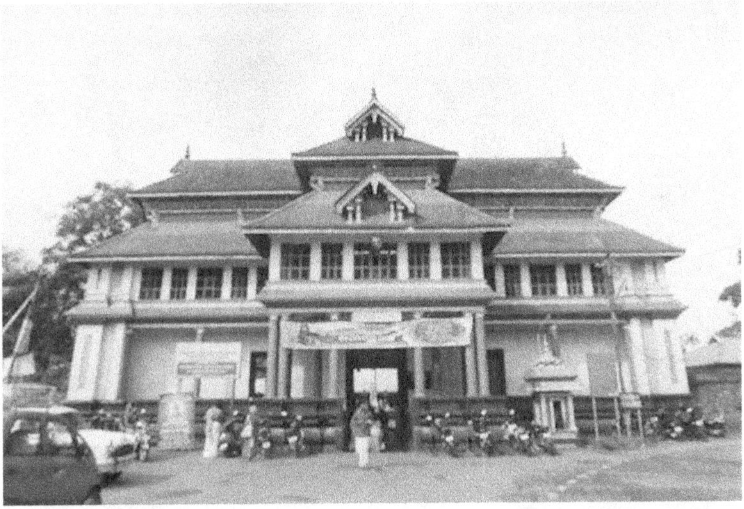

Figure 9: Entrance to the Sree Mahadevar/Bhagavathy temple, Chengannur, 2014

In the small and beautiful town of Chengannur, every person, male included, spoke with pride of the menstrual festival, thriputh-aarattu, to anyone who was a newcomer. My team and I had the opportunity to visit the temple, interact with the temple authorities, devotees, and also meet the parents of the Melśānti[1] of Sabarimala, who does the special pūjā during the thriputh-aarattu. We even got the opportunity of a one-on-one interview with the Melśānti's mother, Smt. Devika Devi, who is the only person allowed to inspect the udayada (inner skirt) of Devī and decide if she is indeed menstruating or not.

When the Melśānti detects a stain on the Devī's udayada, it is brought to Thazhamon Madam, the residence of Smt. Devika Devi, for inspection by her. She informed us that her mother-in-law used to tell her that years ago, Devī's menstruation used to happen every month. However, in recent years, it occurs only

3-4 times annually. It is said that many years ago, Devī used to menstruate for 2-3 days at a time, but now, it is only a few drops on the first day.

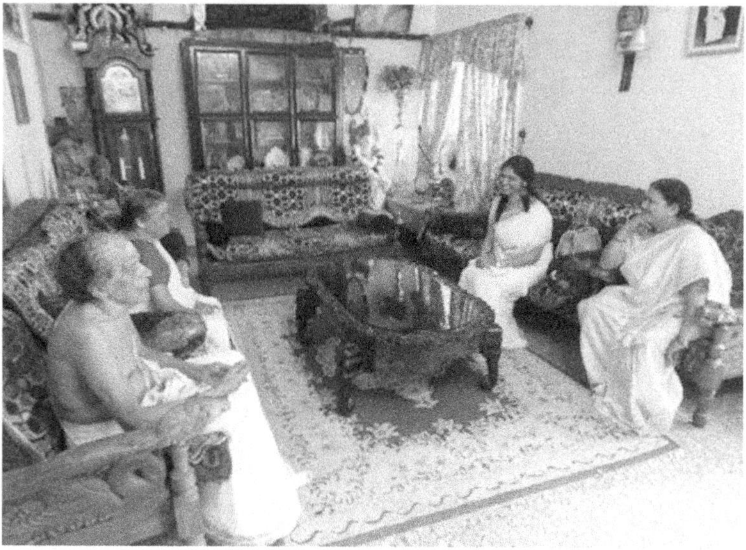

Figure 10: Parents of the Sabarimala Melsanthi (left) in conversation with the author and Mrs. Vyjayanthi Krishnamurthy, at Thazhamon Madam, 2014

Further, the devotees believe that a visit to this temple, and especially praying to Devī Bhagavathi during thriputh-aarattu, will resolve problems associated with fertility, menstruation, and reproductive issues. It is important to know that their belief comes not through legends or someone else's story, but through their own direct experience of improved health after visiting the temple. How do we make sense of this occurrence?

The legends

Every temple has a story that is passed down from generation to generation. It is usually the first thing narrated by the Melśānti when someone enquires about the temple. These stories sound simple enough, but on close examination, we will find that they hold a great many clues as to the nature of the caitanyam in the temple.

This temple is the abode of Śiva and Parvathi Devī (also called Bhagavathy Devī). According to the official story of the temple authorities, Parvathi Devī was believed to have attained menarche in Chengannur, soon after her marriage to Śiva. Her menarche was a cause for celebration at that time, and the same is followed to this day. The rituals followed for the menstruating Devī is very similar to the rituals followed for young girls who attain menarche, and the temple remains closed for three days during Devī's menstruation. There is another legend associated with this temple, which might explain the aspect of menstruation. As per the temple's official website, the story goes thus:

> The place where the Chengannur temple is situated was said to be under the control of Vanghipuzha Thampuran. This place was leased to Nayanaru Pillai. One day, while the maidservant (Kurathi) of Nayanaru Pillai was working in this place, she saw blood coming from a stone on which she was sharpening her weapon. This fact was reported to Nayanaru Pillai and Vanghipuzha Thampuran, who later constructed the present temple on the same spot.

Decoding the legends

Chengannur means land of the red soil. It is situated in the Allapuzha district of Kerala. The district survey report of Minor Minerals of Allapuzha (2016)[2] reports the presence of laterite and laterite soil in the district. The term 'laterite' was coined by the English surgeon Francis Buchanan when he discovered this formation in Kerala, in 1807. In his report, he has mentioned:

> "What I have called indurated clay...is one of the most valuable materials for building. It is diffused in immense masses, without any appearance of stratification and is placed over the granite that forms the basis of Malayala. It is full of cavities and pores and contains a large quantity of iron in the form of red and yellow ochres."

Laterite is a soil and rock type which is rich in iron. It is possible that the 'blood' coming out of the stone was indicative of an underground spring containing the mineral iron. The water from a spring rich in minerals like iron can turn red upon oxidation, resembling blood. Throughout India, we find temples constructed around underground springs rich in minerals, owing to the healing properties of the minerals in the spring. The Kāmākhya temple in Assam, which is famous for the underground spring which turns red once a year, marking the menstruation of Kāmākhya Devī, is another example of such phenomena. That region too is rich in iron content.[3]

If the 'menstrual blood' of Devī is due to the iron content in the underground spring, then it would explain why the inner skirt onto which she bleeds is considered auspicious and booked by devotees months in advance. It is likely that with the environmental damages that Kerala has been witnessing, there has been a depletion of groundwater, and accordingly the frequency of the Devī's menstruation, i.e. the rise in underground spring water, has also been on the decline.

Despite what the facts might be, we must not overlook the aspect of the symbolism, which is as important. The fact that the menstruation of Devī is a celebration in this temple talks volumes of how the Hindu religion and culture honors the menstrual process.

Mr. Munro's wife

The legends and stories about the temple also point to the nature of the caitanyam in the temple. The stories clearly indicate that the caitanyam has something to do with menstruation. One of the earliest stories of women having experienced the caitanyam in this temple and how it impacted their menstrual cycle is described in the story of Mr. Munro. Under the British rule, Sir Thomas Munro, who was the Governor of Madras (16 September 1814 - 10 July 1827), had laughed at the belief that Devī menstruates and stopped all grants for observing her menstrual ritual celebration. Since then, it is said that his wife started bleeding profusely and continuously. Though he supposedly consulted many doctors, his wife's menstrual flow would not stop. A well-wisher of Mr. Munro told him that it may be due to his action of stopping the grants to the Chengannur temple. Mr. Munro then pledged that if his wife is cured, he will create a Trust whose interest would be sufficient to observe the celebration of the thirupoothu (menses) of Devī. His wife is said to have been cured soon after. Apart from creating the Trust, Mr. Munro also presented two golden bangles to Devī. It is said that Mr. Munro's family continues to sponsor the first period of Devī Bhagavathy in Chengannur to date.

Stories such as these are important indicators as to what the caitanyam of the temple is like. It reminds me of one of the women in a workshop I conducted, who had shared her experience. She narrated how her husband would come home early from work on the days she menstruates, just to take her to a temple and prove that the regulations are all nonsense! When asked about any physical problem during menstruation, she mentioned experiencing abdominal cramps but did not think it had anything to do with the temple visit. It is not unlikely that Mr. Munro did the same with his wife, and the consequence was that the apāna vāyu was triggered to such an extent that the bleeding would not stop.

Our conversations with devotees and temple authorities helped us understand the strong belief people have in the power of the menstruating Devī. Many people are believed to have been cured of problems of infertility and menstrual issues by praying to Bhagwathi Devī during thriputh-aarattu. Yet, the temple has the usual regulation for the entry of menstruating women. It is one thing to have the apāna vāyu regulated when a woman is not menstruating. It is quite another to trigger the already active apāna while a woman is menstruating.

My experience

This temple was an important turning point in my understanding of how ancient Hindu temples impact menstrual health. And the reason was my own experience.

After my return from this temple, there was an unusual shift in my menstrual cycle. It shifted by 13 days, which has never before happened to me. When I sought the help of Jayant ji, who has been guiding my studies of this nature, to understand this shift, he pointed out that the change in date has made my cycle come closer to the earth's fertility cycle. The shift made my period come closer to amāvāsyā or the new moon day in the following months. The significance of this shift wasn't clear to me at first. I later learned that traditionally, it was understood that women who menstruate around the time of amāvāsyā and ovulate around the time of pūrṇimā (full moon) have better reproductive health.

I visited the same temple a year later, and again, my menstrual cycle altered, but in a very different manner. My second visit coincided with the Sabarimala season. The Chengannur Bhagavathy temple lies on the bank of the river Pampa, and it is one of the stops for the Ayyappa devotees on the way to Sabarimala. Ayyappa devotees are required to undertake a 41-day pilgrimage with several rules and regulations that are meant to put them on the path of spirituality. The pilgrimage of Ayyappa devotees and the Sabarimala shrine are designed to take the devotee closer to mokṣa. One of the rules of the pilgrimage is that Ayyappa devotees maintain a physical distance from women in the menstruating age.

On the day of my second visit to the Chengannur Bhagavathy temple, hundreds of Ayyappa devotees had crowded the temple. They were everywhere and made it impossible to even go near the shrine. We had to content ourselves from a distance and left after taking a few interviews with the Melśānti and Smt. Devika Devi. It was during this interview that she told me of how visiting Sabarimala can affect the health of women in the reproductive age and that is the reason for the regulation. The very next day after my return from Chengannur, I got my period, one week before the expected date. This was very unusual, and it threw my cycle totally out of sync.

It is likely that the Ayyappa devotees' presence impacted my cycle. It is perhaps for good reason that Ayyappa devotees are asked to stay away from women, and vice versa, during the time of their 41-day pilgrimage[4]. If the presence of the devotees alone can have such an impact on menstrual cycles, imagine what Sabarimala itself can do to women in the reproductive age.

When we attempt to study temples, it is too easy to get caught up in the legend, the stories, and the symbolism. But if we limit it to merely explaining the symbolism, it would be a case of missing the forest for the trees. We must not forget that the stories and legends point to the underlying caitanyam and provide important clues as to what its nature is like.

This much was clear to me—at a physiological level, spaces like the Bhagavathy temple in Chengannur are capable of shifting women's cycles to align it with nature's cycles, thereby fixing the menstrual and reproductive health of women who enter that space. Verifying this is only a matter of experiencing it.

References for Chapter 9

1. The word Melśānti is the Malayalam word for pūjāri which refers to the person who officiates the rituals and offerings in a Hindu temple. The other words are paṇḍit, purohit, etc.

2. District Survey Report of Minor Minerals (Except Sand River), Allapuzha District, prepared as per Environment Impact Assessment (EIA) Notification, 2006 issued under Environment (Protection) Act 1986 by Department of Mining and Geology

3. When it comes to minerals in springs and their medicinal benefits, Japan is known for propagating their medicinal springs as spas and bathing facilities known as Onsen. Based on the mineral in the spring, the color of the water and the medicinal quality varies, and is common knowledge in Japan. For ex., springs rich in Sulphur are milky white in color and are popular for curing lifestyle diseases, joint aches and skin problem. Similarly, springs which are rich in Iron have a brownish-red color and are popular as springs for women, owing to their medicinal properties for curing anemia and menstrual disorders, among other illnesses. Examples of such iron rich springs in Japan are Noboribetsu Onsen (Hokkaido), Sukaya Onsen (Tohoku region), Arima Onsen (Osaka Kyoto Kansai Region), etc.

4. Joseph, Sinu. Women & Sabarimala: Science behind restriction. Notion Press, 2019

CHAPTER 10

MANTRAS AND THEIR EFFECT ON MENSTRUAL CYCLES

Mantras are the recitation of Saṃskṛtam words and sounds that are known to invoke certain powers, fulfill wishes, grant good health, promote well-being, and in some cases, attain mokṣa, much like the effect of ancient Hindu temples on human beings. Like temples, mantras also act by energizing cakras, thereby impacting the human system.

Mantra Vidyā is a science in itself that needs to be thoroughly understood in order to appreciate how a mantra can manifest the intention for which it is uttered. While it is beyond the scope of this book to elaborate on this science, some existing works offer simplified explanations presented below.

It is said in Tantra Śāstra that the pañcamahābhūtas were produced in the order of ākāśa (ether), vāyu (air), agni (fire), āpā (water), and pṛthvi (earth). From these issued the ṣat-cakras (six cakras), which are said to correspond to each of the pañcamahābhūta, with the ājñā and viśuddhi cakra corresponding to ākāśa (ether), anāhata cakra to vāyu (air), maṇipūra cakra to agni (fire), svadhiṣṭhāna cakra to jal (water), and mūlādhāra cakra to pṛthvi (earth). In Swami Purnananda's work Sat-Cakra-Nirupana, we find that each of the six cakras is

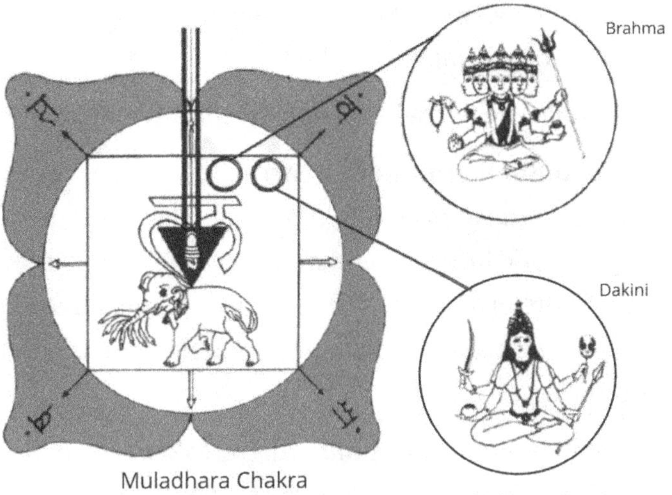

Figure 11: Mūlādhāra Cakra
(Source: Swami Sivananda Radha, Kundalini Yoga for the West, copyright 2005timelessbooks)

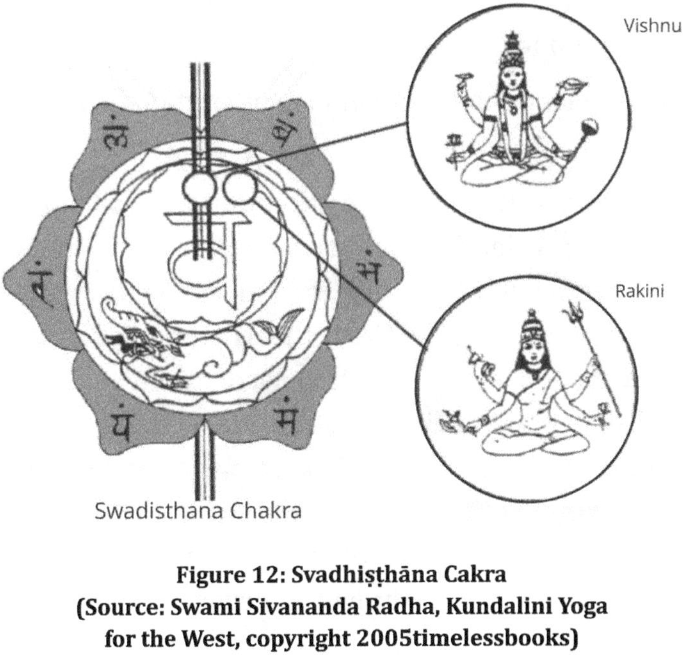

Figure 12: Svadhiṣṭhāna Cakra
(Source: Swami Sivananda Radha, Kundalini Yoga for the West, copyright 2005timelessbooks)

represented as a lotus, with the petals having the alphabets of the Saṃskṛtam language.

In his book The Serpent Power, Sir John Woodroffe writes[1]:

"The total number of petals corresponds with the number of letters of the Saṃskṛtam alphabet. The number of petals of any specific lotus is determined by the disposition of the subtle nāḍīs around it. These petals, further bear specific sound-powers and are fifty in number, as are the letters of the Saṃskṛtam alphabet."

In the representation of mūlādhāra cakra above, there are four petals, representing the Saṃskṛtam letters va, śa, ṣ, sa and the sounds vam, śam, ṣam, sam. Svadhiṣṭhāna cakra has six petals, representing the letters ba, bha, ma, ya, ra, la and the sounds bam, bham, mam, yam, ram, lam. Similarly, the other four cakras are also co-related with particular Saṃskṛtam letters and sounds.

A more elaborate explanation is offered in the book Shakti and Shakta by Woodroffe[2]:

"The letters are (with the exception next stated) placed in the cakras in the alphabetical order; that is, the vowels as being the first letters or Śakti of the consonants (which cannot be produced without them) are placed in Viśuddhi cakra, the first consonants from ka to tha in Anāhata, and so forth until the Mūlādhāra wherein are set the last four letters from va to sa. Thus, in ājñā there are ha and kṣa as being Brahma bīja. In the next, Viśuddhi, are the 16 vowels which originated first. Therefore, they are placed in Viśuddhi, the ethereal cakra, ether having originated first. The same principle applies to the other letters in the cakras, namely, ka to tha (12 letters and petals) in Anāhata; da to pha (10) in Maṇipūra, ba to la (6) in Svadhiṣṭhāna, va to sa (4) in Mūlādhāra. The connection between particular letters and the cakras in which they are placed is further said to be due to the fact that in uttering any particular letter, the cakra in which it is placed and its surroundings are brought into play. The sounds of the Saṃskṛtam alphabet are classified according to the organs used in their articulation, and are guttural (kaṇṭha), palatals (tālu), ceberals (mūrddhā), dentals (danta) and labials (oṣṭha). When so articulated, each letter, it is said "touches" the cakra in which it is, and in which on this account it has been placed."

What this essentially means is that reciting certain mantras can have a specific impact on the person, based on the cakras which are triggered by that particular mantra's sounds. At times, attempts are made to translate a mantra to understand its meaning. While there is no harm in doing so, the true experience of a mantra is not in its verbal meaning but on the impact the sounds have on the physical and subtle body. This is the reason why Saṃskṛtam scholars give tremendous importance to correct pronunciation; the meanings are secondary.

Similar to the effect of temples, even with mantras, unless they energize the lower cakras, they could cause problems in women's reproductive health. This is explained below with the example of the ancient Gayatri Mantra, which, as per its original version in Ṛgveda, is not recommended for women in the menstrual age.

The ancient Gayatri Mantra

Gayatri Mantra is a 6,000-year-old verse recited by millions of Hindus every day. This mantra (Ṛgveda Saṃhitā 3.62.10) was composed by Sage Vishwamitra. Ideally, the sacred Gayatri Mantra should be recited, comprehended, and studied only by those who have been initiated for this. For this reason, I will not be going into the description of the mantra itself and will only focus on its impact on women's bodies. The original Gayatri Mantra, as mentioned in the Ṛgveda, consists of the following lines:

तत्सवितुर्वरेण्यं
भर्गो देवस्य धीमहि
धियो यो नः प्रचोदयात्

tat-savitur vareṇyaṃ
bhargo devasya dhīmahi
dhiyo yo naḥ prachodayāt

But the version that is recited today has the addition of ॐ भूर्भुवः स्वः (om bhūr bhuvaḥ svaḥ) to the beginning of the Gayatri Mantra. While om is the prāṇava[3] which is recited at the start of all mantras, the other three sounds are called vyāhṛti. The three vyāhṛtis are added at the beginning of the original Gayatri Mantra, for a reason which will be explained later in this chapter.

The original Gayatri Mantra, without the introductory vyāhṛti, is generally not recommended for women in the reproductive age as per the ancient rules. This mantra is said to cause reproductive disorders in women and results in women developing masculine features such as excessive facial hair, deepened masculine voice, and infertility. With the knowledge of cakras, it is possible to explain how this mantra works on human physiology and why these regulations exist.

Impact on the reproductive system

Mantras are the subtle sounds that activate specific cakras. The Gayatri Mantra in its original form activates the ājñā cakra (located between the eyebrows) and the corresponding pituitary gland. The hypothalamus and pituitary gland play an important role in the reproductive process of both men and women.

In adult males and females, the hypothalamic pulsatile secretion of the gonadotropin-releasing hormone (GnRH) results in the expression and release of follicle-stimulating hormone (FSH) and luteinizing hormone (LH) from the anterior pituitary gland. FSH and LH (gonadotropins) regulate the function of the testes and ovaries (gonads). [4]

In men, LH stimulates testosterone production from the interstitial cells of the testes. So, an activated ājñā cakra in men corresponds to a well-functioning pituitary gland and the production of testosterone. Similarly, in women, LH stimulates testosterone production in the ovary. Unlike men, however, women must have much lower concentrations of testosterone, and it only rises at the time around ovulation. In women, testosterone is important for muscle strength as well as to increase sexual libido necessary for procreation. The female hormone estrogen is made from testosterone and other adrenal hormones. Without the ability of women's bodies to make testosterone, they cannot make estrogen. Estrogen is what causes ovulation, followed by menstruation.

The impact of Gayatri Mantra on the female body is explained by Jayant ji in the below passage from his write-up[5]:

> "The female physical body manifests capability to pro-create and nurture. To activate these capabilities, it draws upon the energies of the Mūlādhāra, Svadhiṣṭhāna, Maṇipūra and Anāhata.
>
> Vibrational mantras (set apart from contemplative mantras) are practiced to activate specific energy centers. The Gayatri mantra is a vibrational mantra, practiced to activate the Ājñā energy, to enable access to analytical intelligence.
>
> Practice of the Gayatri mantra on a daily basis over a sustained period of time may lead to more energy channeled towards analytical (Ājñā) actions and relatively less energy towards survival (Mūlādhāra) and pro-creative (Svadhiṣṭhāna) actions. The Viśuddhi expressions may also be more analytical and less compassionate and nurturing, by those practicing the Gayatri.
>
> The Gayatri mantra practice, therefore, may not make sense to be practiced for those with female bodies, who wish to be mostly active in pro-creation and compassionate nurturing."

Regular chanting of the original Gayatri Mantra by women triggers the ājñā cakra but ignores the svadhiṣṭhāna and mūlādhāra cakras, causing the ovaries to eventually become dysfunctional. The release of hormones is influenced by a feedback loop from the ovaries during the menstrual cycle in a healthy female. Under ordinary circumstances, increased level of hormones inhibits GnRH production through a negative feedback loop. However, in the case of dysfunctional ovaries, such feedback does not happen, resulting in the pituitary producing excess LH. Once the ovaries become dysfunctional, there will be inadequate production of estrogen by the ovaries, resulting in excess testosterone.

While an increase in testosterone is not harmful to men, even a slight increase in testosterone in a woman's body can suppress normal menstruation and/or ovulation. The resulting symptoms of excess testosterone might be the cause for such women to have male characteristics of excessive facial hair (hirsutism), deepened masculine voice, and difficulty reproducing.

Hypothalamic-pituitary-ovarian axis

The hypothalamic-pituitary-ovarian (HPO) axis is a tightly regulated system controlling female reproduction. HPO axis dysfunction leading to ovulation disorders can be classified into three categories defined by the World Health Organization (WHO). Group I ovulation disorders involve hypothalamic failure characterized as hypogonadotropic hypogonadism. Group II disorders display a eugonadal state commonly associated with a wide range of endocrinopathies. Finally, Group III constitutes hypergonadotropic hypogonadism secondary to depleted ovarian function. [6]

Group II eugonadal ovulatory dysfunction accounts for the majority of ovulation disorders and comprises a wide spectrum of disorders, including PCOS. Polycystic ovary syndrome (PCOS) is the most common endocrine disorder in reproductive age women and a common cause for anovulation. Few of the mechanisms describing the pathogenesis of PCOS include loss of GnRH pulsatility with increased LH secretion by the pituitary gland, hyperinsulinemia, ovarian insulin resistance, theca cell dysfunction, and hyperandrogenism.[9]

Group III ovulatory disorders are defined as ovarian insufficiency or failure with a hypergonadotrophic-hypogonadic profile that affects 5% of women with ovulatory dysfunction.[8] Early depletion of ovarian function before the age of 40, associated with elevated FSH or low estradiol levels, is defined as premature ovarian insufficiency (POI), formerly known as premature ovarian failure.[9]

Some of the symptoms of Group II and Group III ovulatory disorders are similar to what is described as the impact of continuously energizing only the ājña cakra. It is possible that continuous chanting of the original Gayatri Mantra by women in the reproductive age might result in PCOS or POI and associated menstrual and reproductive difficulties.

Gayatri Mantra as recited today

But, how is it that many women today chant the Gayatri Mantra, without experiencing the above-mentioned effects? This is where the role of the vyāhṛti comes into play.

The vyāhṛtis were believed to be made at the beginning of creation and represent the seven planetary systems, viz., Bhūr, Bhuva, Svāhā, Mahah, Janah, Tapah, and Satyalokas. Besides denoting the seven worlds, the vyāhṛtis denote the seven planes of consciousness and also the cakras. The seven vyāhṛtis are seven invocations which invoke the cakras as follows[10]:

1. Bhūr - Physical - Mūlādhāra
2. Bhuva - Vital - Svadhiṣṭhāna
3. Svāhā - Mental - Maṇipūra

4. Mahah - Intellectual - Anāhata
5. Janah - Super mental - Viśuddhi
6. Tapah - Spiritual - Ājñā
7. Satyam - Absolute reality – Sahasrāra

Therefore, in the version of the Gayatri Mantra recited today, the three sounds following om help to balance the mantra because bhūr activates the mūlādhāra cakra, bhuva activates the svadhiṣṭhāna cakra, and svāhā activates the maṇipūra cakra. When these vyāhṛtis are added to the original Gayatri Mantra, it is not just the activation of the ājñā cakra, but also of the three lower cakras, which are essential for women in the reproductive age. This creates a balancing effect and makes it suitable for women in the menstruating age as well.

A note about OM chanting for women

The sacred universal sound of OM, when chanted with the sounds 'O' and 'M', energize the higher cakras from the region of the chest to the head. We can experience this in the form of reverberations in the said regions while chanting OM. Since this version of OM chanting only energizes the higher cakras, it is generally not recommended for women in the reproductive age.

Whereas, when it is chanted as AUM, with the sounds 'A', 'U', and 'M', it also activates the lower cakras. When chanted as A-U-M, we can experience the reverberations from the pelvic area all the way up to the head. Hence, it is recommended that women in the reproductive age group should chant AUM instead of OM.

The easiest way to understand a mantra's effect is simply by uttering it with regularity in the form of a sādhana and observing the impact it brings about. This is the way in which our ancestors understood complex phenomena—through their sādhana and the resulting experience.

References for Chapter 10

1. Avalon, Arthur (Sir John Woodroffe). The Serpent Power: The Secrets of Tantric and Shaktic Yoga, 1919
2. Woodrooffe, Sir John. Shakti and Shakta, Sec 3, Chap. Shakti as Mantra, 1929
3. Prāṇava is the primordial sound that existed before creation. Every mantra starts with Om.
4. Gonadotropin Releasing Hormone. Sepideh Khazeni, Pegah Varamini, in Reference Module in Biomedical Sciences, 2018
5. Kalawar, Jayant. The Feminine and Masculine in Each of Us: Dancing with our Cakras. Feb 2017, www.21banyantree.com
6. Mikhael S, Punjala-Patel A, Gavrilova-Jordan L. Hypothalamic-Pituitary-Ovarian Axis Disorders Impacting Female Fertility. Biomedicines. 2019;7(1):5. Published 2019 Jan 4.
7. Legro R.S., Arslanian S.A., Ehrmann D.A., Hoeger K.M., Murad M.H., Pasquali R., Welt C.K., Society E. Diagnosis and treatment of polycystic ovary syndrome: An Endocrine Society clinical practice guideline. J. Clin. Endocrinol. Metab. 2013;98:4565–4592.
8. O'Flynn N. Assessment and treatment for people with fertility problems: NICE guideline. Br. J. Gen. Pract. 2014;64:50–51.
9. Legro R.S., Arslanian S.A., Ehrmann D.A., Hoeger K.M., Murad M.H., Pasquali R., Welt C.K., Society E. Diagnosis and

treatment of polycystic ovary syndrome: An Endocrine Society clinical practice guideline. J. Clin. Endocrinol. Metab. 2013;98:4565–4592.

10. This information has been taken from the article on Vedamata Gayatri from this source - www.kamakotimandali.com/srividya/vedamata.html

Chapter 11

Kāmākhya: Where Menstruation Meets Spirituality

The Kāmākhya temple in Guwahati, Assam, is popular as the temple where Devī Kāmākhya is believed to menstruate for four days, every year. Her menstruation is a major celebration in the region, during which time all temples, businesses, and farming activities in the region are paused. Everyone rests, as the Great Mother Kāmākhya herself is considered to be resting during her annual menstrual phase. These four days are celebrated as a festival called Ambubachi, which usually happens between June $21^{st}/22^{nd}$ to June $24^{th}/25^{th}$.

The association of Kāmākhya with menstruation made it one of the key places to be visited on my list. My first visit was in March 2015. The positive reinforcement of menstruation in the culture and traditions of this region become obvious when we visit this place. It gives us a clue of how menstruation was originally revered in this land. Apart from the Chengannur Bhagavathy temple in Kerala, this was the other place where one could find men queuing up for a piece of the Devī's auspicious menstrual cloth. But the scale of celebration here is something else. In 2019, when I visited here the second time, there were around 25 lakh devotees during the four days of Ambubachi!

There are a great many fascinating stories about this temple, and each one of those stories will take us in circles. The play of māyā [1] here is such that we will feel that we know a lot about this temple, but in reality, we would not have understood even a grain of truth about Ma Kāmākhya. She is a very bewildering entity, and only through her own grace can one learn anything about her. This place requires us to drop our scholarly hat, and simply submit to Her Will.

Too many questions, too few answers

I would have forgotten all about my first visit in March 2015, except that for two years since my visit, the first day of my period in the month of June coincided exactly with the first day of Ambubachi (22nd June 2016 and 22nd June 2017). While my hectic work schedule threw my cycles out of sync in 2018, I was back on track the following year, and it happened again on 21st June 2019, the year I undertook my second visit to write this book. And again, it happened on 21st June 2020 when I made the final edits to this book. She simply wouldn't let me forget.

This prompted my first series of questions – Why did my period coincide with Ambubachi four times? Can four times even be called a coincidence? And what does it mean that the Devī 'menstruates'?

If we try to answer these questions through the symbolism in Kāmākhya, we will be even more bewildered. After all, this is a rare temple where there is no mūrti of the Devī in the sanctum. She is represented as a yōni[2]. The temple is a natural cave and the underground sanctum has a natural stone formation which slopes on either side, looking very much like a yōni. There is a perennial underground spring that keeps the yōni moist all year through. The length of the yōni is almost 1.5 ft in length and 1 ft in breadth.[3] During Ambubachi, the water from her yōni is said to turn red. But we cannot see the change in color because the doors of the sanctum remain closed until Ambubachi is over. During the days when it is open, devotees are allowed to enter the sanctum and offer prayers, touching the yōni and the water therein, unlike in most temples where the sanctum is off-limits for devotees. In fact, I saw devotees fill the water in bottles and drink from it, as it is said to cure all kinds of problems. A piece of cloth moistened by this water is the prized possession that devotees are willing to pay thousands of rupees for, though it was not officially sold at the time of my visit.

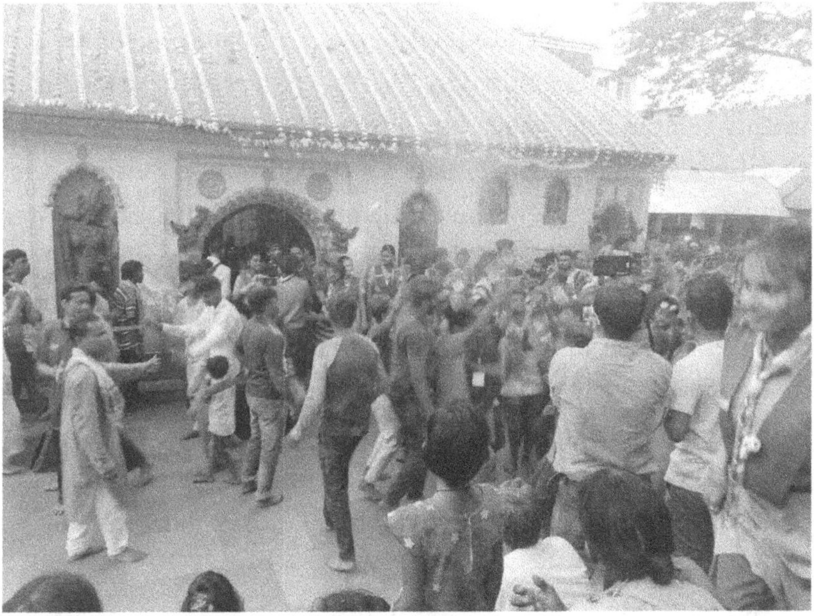

Figure 13: Men celebrating the menstruation of Devī Kāmakhya, June 26, 2019

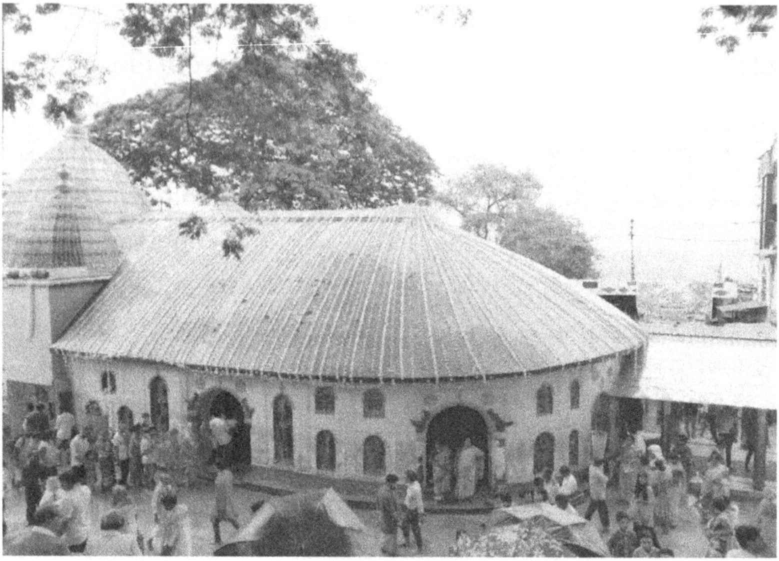

Figure 14: Kāmakhya temple decorated for Ambubachi, June 26, 2019

The legend associated with this temple is also a little unusual. If we ask people why the Devī is represented as a yōni in this temple, they will typically narrate the story of Sati's[4] sacrifice. As per the lore, Sati sacrificed her body in a duel between her father Daksha and her husband Śiva. Seeing her dead, Śiva lost his mind and carried her corpse around in great grief, not able to bear the pain of her death. Unable to bear Śiva's grief, Vishnu thought it best to chop Sati's body with his disc, forcing Śiva to let go of it. From the parts of Sati's body that fell in different places on earth, the 52 Śakti Pīṭhas came into being. These Śakti Pīṭhas are the key places for experiencing Śakti. The part of Sati's body which fell in Kāmākhya is said to be the yōni.

But the Kāmākhya temple is not the only temple where the Devī is represented as the yōni. In the same hill where she resides, called Nilachal, there are temples of the Daśa Mahā Vidyās, which refers to the ten great sources of wisdom, with each being represented as a Devī. In these temples too, the sanctum has the yōni representing each of the Daśa Mahā Vidyās, namely Kāli, Tāra, Tripurasundarī, Bhuvaneśvarī, Bhairavī, Chinnamasta, Dhūmavati, Bagalamukhī, Mātaṅgī, and Kamala.[19] These temples too remain closed during Ambubachi.

There is a norm that before visiting Ma Kāmākhya, devotees must first pay respects to and seek permission from Śrī Umānanda at the Umānanda temple. This temple of Śiva as Umānanda is located in the river island of Brahmaputra, about 8 km from the Kāmākhya temple. The paṇḍit also informed us that only after the darśan of Ma Kāmākhya should one visit other Daśa Mahā Vidyās, and never the other way around. This leads to the next set of questions:

- Why should one visit the Umānanda temple first?
- Since there is no mūrti of Kāmākhya, how should one understand who she is?

Sometimes described as Kāli, sometimes as Sati, sometimes as Umānanda's Uma, sometimes as Kāmeshwari who satisfies all desires, and sometimes as the Daśa Mahā Vidyās; who exactly is Ma Kāmākhya?

The other surprising polarity we see here is the contrast of devotees that Ma Kāmākhya attracts. On one hand, the Ambubachi festival sees a host of Tantrics[5] and other ascetics camping in the temple premises for four days, all in an effort to complete their sādhana of spiritual realization and merging with Brahman. The time when Ma Kāmākhya menstruates is said to be ideal for this purpose.

On the other hand, we see lakhs of common men and women, across castes and class, who come here for fulfilling their many desires of worldly life. And the strange part is that all devotees are said to experience fulfillment of their wishes in this place. In other words, be it the pursuit of mukti (spiritual liberation) or bhukti (worldly pleasure), all wishes are granted in the abode of Ma Kāmākhya. She is said to be the one who fulfills all desires and ensures mukti as well.

Does this not seem contradictory? Yet, there are no contradictions. Only our lack of understanding.

Decoding Ambubachi

In June 2019, I had planned my travels in such a way that I would complete touring Sabarimala's four temples[6] and then come back home to rest during menstruation (which coincided with Ambubachi) and then set off to Kāmākhya when the temple opens just after the festival. Ambubachi is celebrated on the seventh to the eleventh day of the lunar month of āṣāḍha, as per the lunar Bengali calendar, and usually occurs between June 22nd to June 25th every year. On June 25th, 2019, I reached Guwahati a day before the temple was to be opened.

The summer heat was at its peak on that day. If you went outdoors, you could feel the heat rising from the ground below. The locals expressed that the rains ought to come, but had not yet arrived. But the very next day, when the Kāmākhya temple opened, the sky burst forth and it rained heavily. Monsoon had arrived perfectly in time when Mother Kāmākhya and Mother Earth's menstruation had ended. Without a doubt, the celebration and recognition of Kāmākhya's menstruation were intrinsically connected to the understanding of the earth's annual menstrual cycle. The lunar months of jyeṣṭhā and āṣāḍha (around mid-May to mid-July) together make the Indian season of Grīṣma kāla or summer. This is the time when all beings experience internal thermoregulation. This is the season when the pañcamahābhūtas of agni and vāyu, and as a result, pitta doṣa and vāta doṣa, are at an all-time high, and consequently, a menstruation-like environment is created. But this is not just symbolic. It has an impact on human menstrual cycles as well.

It is probably no coincidence that Ambubachi starts a day after the summer solstice, which falls on June 21st. This is the time when the sun reaches its highest position in the sky; consequently, June 21st is the hottest and longest day of the year in India. The state of Assam in North-Eastern India was originally called Pragjyotiṣapura, which literally meant 'ancient place in the East of the science of light/astrology/astronomy'. This name was probably in acknowledgment of this region experiencing this effect in a profound way. While I was there, I simply could not get used to bright sunlight at 3:00 A.M which resembles the sunlight at around 6.30 A.M in South India, where I live.

Women in reasonably good health will be able to notice that just before the phase of Dakṣiṇāyana[7] starts after the summer solstice, their menstrual cycles will undergo a shift. If the menstrual cycle was occurring close to the new moon before the summer solstice, it will shift closer to the full moon after the solstice, and vice versa. This major shift from uttarāyaṇa to dakṣiṇāyana, marked by Mother Earth's menstrual phase, is what is culturally represented in Kāmākhya temple through the Ambubachi festival. It serves as a reminder to women to observe their own cycles and pay attention to the shifts in nature. Visiting the Kāmākhya temple helps women come in sync with nature's larger cycles, thereby restoring our health and vitality. And that is probably why my menstrual date in June began syncing with Ambubachi.

Umānanda Temple

We decided to follow the rule book and visit the Umānanda temple one day before we set foot in Kāmākhya. Ideally, both the temples should be visited on the same day, but owing to the large number of devotees at Kāmākhya temple, we had to do it over two days. The Umānanda temple, dedicated to Śiva, is located in a river island of the Brahmaputra river. This island is considered as the world's smallest inhabited river island. To reach this temple, it is necessary to take a ferry service from the mainland, which takes only about 10 minutes to reach the island. The temple is surrounded by lush greenery and looks deceivingly simple.

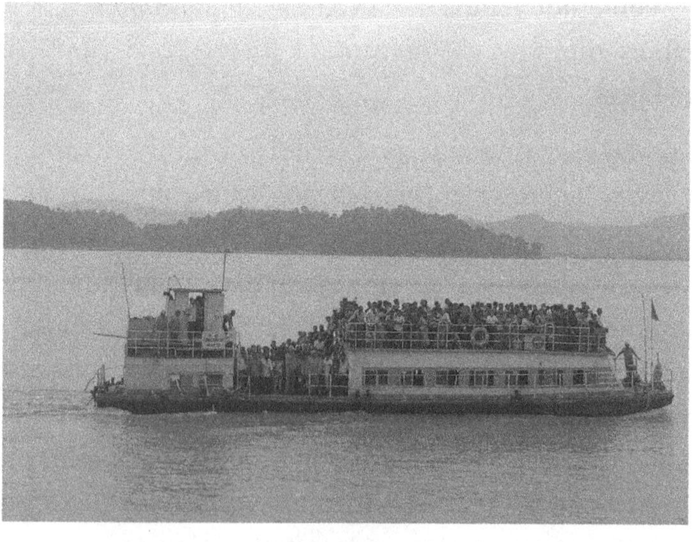

Figure 15: Government-operated ferry service to the Umānanda Temple

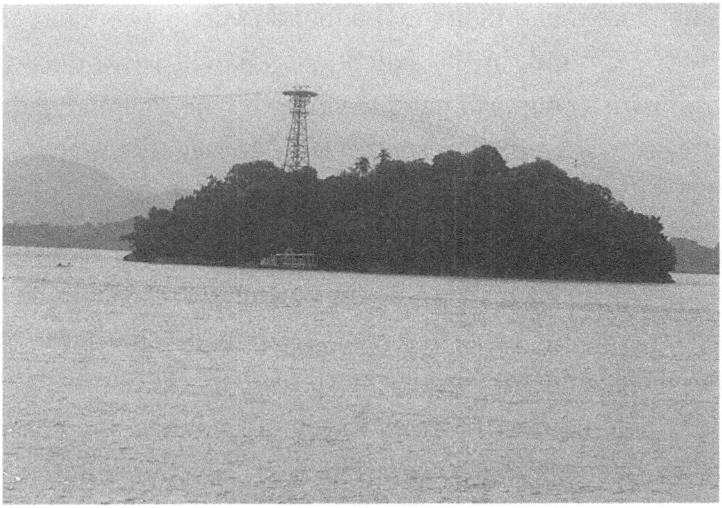

Figure 16: The island in river Brahmaputra, where Umānanda Temple is situated

The ferry had loudspeakers blaring out 90s Bollywood songs, which had the power to give anyone a headache. The people who were with us during the ferry ride were a noisy bunch—chatting, fighting, taking selfies, and singing Bollywood songs all along the route as if they were on a picnic, rather than a visit to a temple. As much as I tried to go into a meditative silence and prepare myself for whatever the temple beholds, it was impossible to do so, with all the noise and distraction. But when this same crowd started to descend the steps to the sanctum, an eerie silence followed. Everyone just went still, as though they could not help it. A very powerful presence permeated the temple, which was felt by all who were present. Suddenly, a group of devotees started making a tribal hooting sound by tapping their mouths with their hands, making us feel like we were going to witness something very sacred and unusual. As I realized in retrospect, that feeling was not wrong.

The main sanctum in the Umānanda temple was a few steps below the ground. In the sanctum, we could see a decorated trishul[8] with a couple of paṇḍits sitting by the side of it, guiding devotees to offer their respects. Here too, unlike many other temples, devotees were allowed into the sanctum.

Just before taking the first step to the descent, my eyes fell upon an engraving on brass at the entrance of the stairs. It was unmistakably the image of Rudra, the deity in Maṇipūra Cakra! In the diagrammatic representation of the Maṇipūra Cakra, there is a depiction of Śiva as Rudra in the form of an ascetic, with ash smeared all over him, sitting in tapas (meditation).

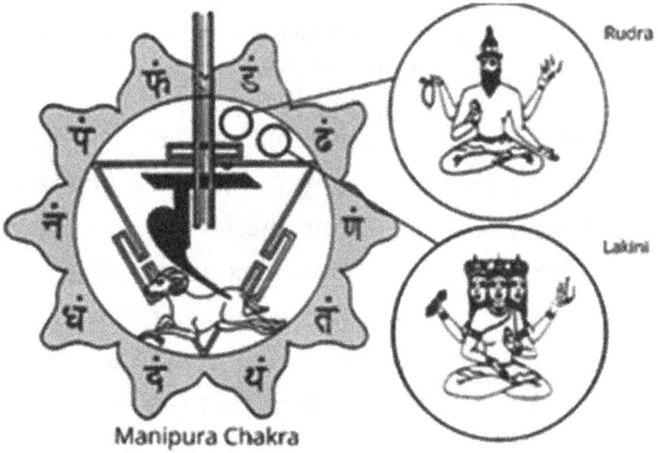

Figure 17: Manipura Chakra
(Source: Swami Sivananda Radha, Kundalini Yoga for the West, copyright 2005timelessbooks)

Before this could even sink in mentally, the crowd started to descend toward the sanctum, and I too was pushed along with the others. As we got closer, I felt a very obvious throbbing in the entire region of the solar plexus, in almost a straight line, making me realize that this is the region of the maṇipūra cakra. It was so tangible that if someone put their hand over my abdomen, I was certain that they could also feel the pulsations. With this throbbing feeling, I reached the sanctum and bent down to offer my respects in silence, when the paṇḍit suddenly thudded my back, quite heavily, twice, and said something to bless me. He did this to everyone who bent down. If you were unprepared like me, it will leave you somewhat shaken.

Nothing in this place is subtle. If one does not feel the throbbing in the maṇipūra cakra naturally, the paṇḍit will make sure that he beats it into activation! Bhaskar, who accompanied me on this visit, agreed that he too felt similar sensations in the abdominal region. This place triggered the maṇipūra cakra; we could feel it in a very perceptible way. It was so powerful a feeling that it did not go away and remained even the next morning when we had to visit the Kāmākhya temple.

The legend of the Umānanda temple offers clues as to why it is important to visit here before going to the Kāmākhya temple. The site of this temple is the spot where Śiva, during meditation, was disturbed by Kāmadeva, the Deva of love and desire. Śiva, in his anger, burned Kāmadeva to ashes (bhasm) and so this hill got the name Bhasmāchala.

The maṇipūra cakra, with the ascetic attributes of Rudra operating at the region of the solar plexus (abdomen), is often considered as the stepping stone to the higher cakras, enabling devotees to develop vairāgya (detachment) toward worldly life. We can experience this in the Sabarimala temple tradition as well, where the Aryankavu temple of Dharma Shastha in Kollam, Kerala, also works on the maṇipūra cakra, which puts devotees of Swamy Ayyappa on the path of vairāgya and spirituality.[9]

Kāma is the word that denotes worldly desire. The Kāmākhya temple is so powerful in granting desires that devotees can easily get carried away with worldly desires and the vices they bring. To balance this aspect of Kāmākhya, it is recommended to visit the Umānanda temple first, so that unwary devotees are not swept away in the pursuit of Kāma.

Ma Kāmākhya's will

It is said that until and unless Ma Kāmākhya desires it, devotees will not be able to have her darśan. The day the temple opened, and 2 to 3 days after that, there were serpentine queues and unimaginable crowds. Imagine 25 lakh people trying to reach the small cave sanctum. There were devotees who stood in line a day before the temple opened, slept in the queue, never left it even to eat or relieve themselves, and yet had no luck. We did not even attempt to stand in the queue because we knew that it was pointless. Devotees kept saying that only if Ma Kāmākhya wills, we will get to have the darśan. Besides, it started to become obvious that she makes us work hard for it!

We rented a two-wheeler and followed Google Maps to reach one of the entrances to the temple, which Google indicated to be the fastest route. From this entrance, it was a steep climb up with about 150 stone steps. It looked like some sort of a back-door entry and was different from the entrance I had taken during my visit in 2015. I was keen to visit the temple before breakfast, so the climb was done on an empty stomach early in the morning. It was not the best plan because I began to black out. I needed to pause every few steps because of the dizziness. And finally, when we made it to the top, the security personal refused to let us enter because they had closed this entrance owing to the huge crowds.

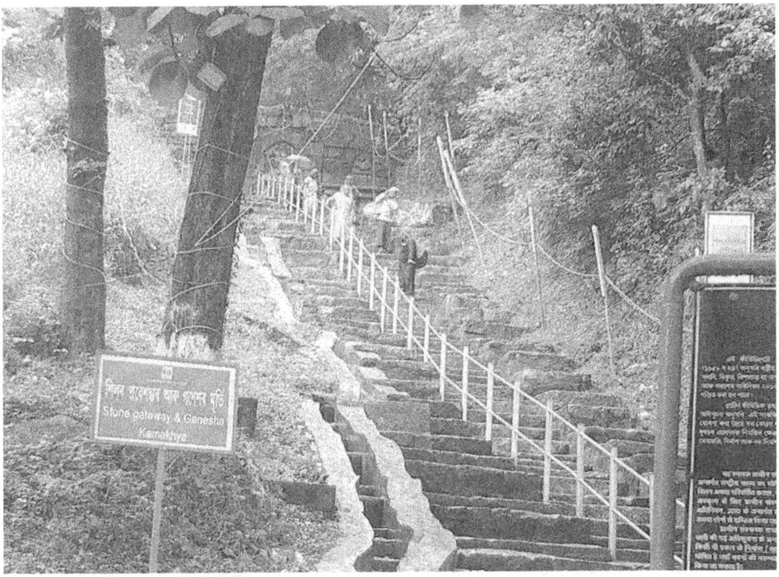

Figure 18: The eastern entrance with steps leading up

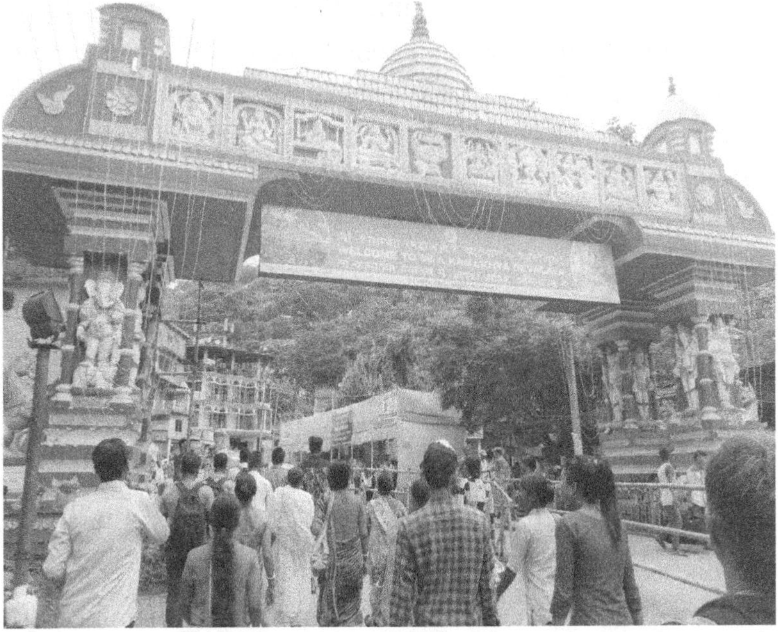

Figure 19: The official western entrance during the Ambubachi

I later learned that this was the eastern entrance, which is for devotees who are seeking mukti. I suppose that explained why most of the people climbing alongside me were sādhus! For those seeking wealth and prosperity, there is another entrance from the western side, which was open to the public during the festive time. I suppose most devotees wouldn't mind the government deciding which entrance is better for them. For others, there is always the strange twist of fate that will put them on the path that they ought to be in.

After being refused entry at the top of the steps, we started to climb back down. All of a sudden, it started to pour wildly, forcing us to stop at some temporary shelter for a couple of hours for the rain to subside. I was exhausted, hungry, disoriented, and very confused. To add to the confusion, there was a tantric, clad in red, frightening people about black magic and how Ma Kāmākhya will punish those who are not following the rules to visit her. People listened to him with fear and awe. Before visiting the Kāmākhya temple, I had heard about black magic being practiced here, and that such people instill fear in devotees to get them to take their services and special pūjā to ward off the evil. I was too weary to feel fear or awe. Meanwhile, everyone who passed by kept suggesting that it is impossible to have the darśan, given the huge crowds.

I was mentally prepared that it would be crowded, but I wasn't prepared for things being so out of hand. Finally, we thought of trying our luck the next day and left to have lunch. But all it took was an hour away, some good lunch, and we felt refreshed. We decided to go back and try entering again from the main entrance on the western side. We made up our mind that no matter how crowded, we will at least remain on the premises, even if we can't have the darśan.

When we entered the temple premises, there was an unmistakable exuberance in the air. Bhaskar put it well, "In this place, everything is amplified." The people are loud, the sounds of animals being sacrificed are loud, the celebrations are very loud, and yet, there is some strange hypnotic effect in the area that will make us go silent in reverence. I was observing how the pigeons were hardly flying around and were just content sitting on the ground, waiting to be picked up to be sacrificed, when suddenly, a side door opened and the guard was looking for devotees who wished to enter. We managed to be among the first in this queue. Although this queue was not going to take us to the sanctum, it did take us for the mūrti darśan, where one can see the mūrti in a hall just before the sanctum entrance. For some reason, I kept hearing it as mukti darśan, which I suppose is not too far from the truth. And so, it began—the experience of Ma Kāmākhya's version of mukti.

Experiencing Kāmākhya

At first, I was too excited to be inside the temple and simply kept looking around for clues as to what this place might be. There were small groups of people undertaking kanya pūjā for their young daughters, aged around 6 to 8 years. There were others sitting in groups in different parts of the temple, undertaking some or the other type of pūjā. I looked around and saw the three-headed Devī Lakini of the maṇipūra cakra, sculpted beautifully against one of the walls. Ṣat-cakra-nirūpaṇa describes Devī Lakini as the fierce Śakti who is fond of meat (māṃsa), and her breast is ruddy with blood and fat which drop from her mouth. She likes to eat cooked rice with dal mixed with meat and blood. She resides in the flesh (māṃsa dhātu). Perhaps it is for her benefit that all the animal sacrifices are being done?

While I was outside, I also noticed the carved images of what seemed like a crocodile on the temple roof and at the door entrances. More specifically, the makara[10], which looks similar to a crocodile, is symbolized in the waters of the svadhiṣṭhāna cakra. The symbols of menstruation and the presence of the yōni itself indicated that this temple was definitely associated with the svadhiṣṭhāna cakra.

As I stood in the queue for the mūrti darśan, I tried to close my eyes and see what was going on inside me. I could feel pulsations in the pit of the stomach, in the abdomen, going in a straight line up and settling with a throbbing feeling at the base of my throat. Unlike my experience in other temples, here the sensations were in too many places, all at once, making it difficult to pinpoint and say that Ma Kāmākhya is this or that. She was everywhere and everything!

As we turned around to return, devotees were picking up various offerings of flowers, kuṅkuma, and just about anything that touched the mūrti, to take home with them. The paṇḍit gave us coins, six of them. The interesting part is that even a week after I returned from Kāmākhya, the coins still carried the vibrations from the place; I could feel the pulsations when I placed them in my palm.

After the mūrti darśan through the closed gate, while returning, we decided to pick a corner inside the temple and simply sit there and observe the inner goings-on. Initially, my focus was wavered, as I kept expecting to be asked to leave, given the crowded nature of the place. But nothing of the sort happened. Nobody bothered us, and we were able to sit inside Kāmākhya temple and meditate for about an hour on the most crowded day of the year! If that isn't Her Will, then I don't know what is.

It was very easy to go into a meditative state here, in spite of the chaos and loud noise all around us. No sooner than five minutes of closing the eyes, we will start to experience sensations very prominently. The place was bursting with vibrations. It was unlike anything I expected. After a while, for me, the sensations settled in one place—the base of my throat. From there, I could feel distinct pulsations in the palate of my mouth, lower lips, and jaws. These were not experiences that came and went. These vibrations lasted even when I occasionally opened my eyes when some child ran into me or had to scoot when someone rushed in with a culled head of an animal to offer to Devī. Meanwhile, Bhaskar had gone so still that there were pigeons resting on his lap!

I understood that what I was feeling was the viśuddhi cakra, located at the base of my throat. But what were those other sensations in and around my mouth? A few weeks later, while reading a book on cakras, I learned that above the viśuddhi, at the root of the palate, is one of the minor cakras called lalanā (also called kalā cakra)[11]. It was interesting that I could experience all of this, without even knowing that such a thing existed.

We returned to the temple the next day as well, waiting for Her Will to shine on us. And again, we were allowed to enter for the mūrti darśan, as the never-ending queue continued to the main sanctum. We decided to sit in our corner and meditate. So, I got a second day to confirm if what I experienced the previous day would repeat. It did repeat in much the same way, but this time in addition to the viśuddhi, I felt as though someone was pressing the space between my eyebrows. A few times, my head fell back because of the force with which the pressing sensation was happening. This was the seat of the ājñā cakra which I now felt, along with the viśuddhi. I was all the more bewildered. How could one feel all of the cakras in one temple? Who indeed was Ma Kāmākhya?

Who is Ma Kāmākhya?

Finally, on the third and last day of our visit, we got a chance to go all the way to the sanctum. The special counter (costing Rs.500 per person) had opened, now that the crowd had somewhat subsided. One of the paṇḍits helped us get tickets, and we stood in line for five hours from 5 A.M to 10 A.M before we managed to enter the sanctum. She does make us work for it!

As we were nearing the sanctum, we first reached the mūrti in the hall. This is the same mūrti whose darśan we had from behind closed gates, the previous two days. But this time, since I was closer, I observed some things that I had previously not noticed. Actually, it was a male devotee standing in front of me who brought my attention to it, when I was trying to keep my eyes closed. He was taller than me and thought I might miss the sight. Despite the crowd, every devotee there not only wants to have the darśan himself but is equally excited about his fellow devotees having the darśan. His insistence made me open my eyes, partly because I feared he might lift me up to give me a better view, as they do with children!

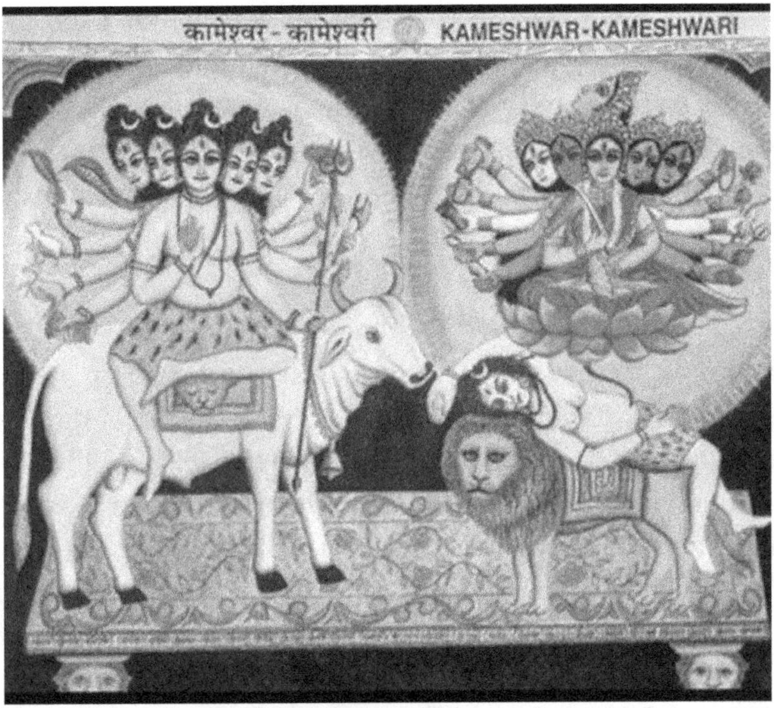

Figure 20:The image of Kameshwar-Kameshwari as seen at Kamakhya temple.

There were three mūrtis, possibly of Ṣoḍaśī, Mātaṅgī, and Kamala, also known as Tripurasundarī, Sarasvatī, and Lakṣmī. Some accounts say that these are the three Devīs who are inside the sanctum, with Ma Kāmākhya. Nearby, I noticed a large framed photograph of Śiva with five faces and ten hands. The image of the five-faced Śiva immediately rang a bell—it was similar to what I have seen of Sadāśiva in the Viśuddhi Cakra's diagrammatic representation. So, that way, I knew that my sensations in the Viśuddhi Cakra were not imaginary. I later learned that Śiva here is known as Kameśwara Śiva. Then there was Devī with six faces and 12 hands, rising from a lotus in the navel of Śiva, who lies inert, like a corpse. This unusual image is what is often used to represent Ma Kāmākhya. There are various interpretations of this image. Some studies say that she is Kameśwari, who is borne by Brahma, Vishnu, and Śiva. The one I like is that Kāmākhya is the creative desire of Śiva. She is his Śakti, created from his desire to express, and taking over from him to create the world.

Kāmākhya in Kāmarūpa

Kāmarūpa in modern-day Assam state is a district. In the ancient days, Kāmarūpa, also called Pragjyotiṣa, was the first historical kingdom in Assam that existed between the 4th to the 12th century CE. [12] The Yogini Tantra describes Kāmarūpa as an important place in a dialogue between Śiva and Pārvati, when she asks him about the chosen place where one can attain siddhi and mukti. In reply to her, Śiva says that japa, homa, etc. become effective when performed in Varanasi,[13] but they yield all the results if performed in Kāmarūpa.[14] Kāmākhya is said to be the center of all sacred places and Devī Kāmākhya is said to reside in every house in Kāmarūpa.

E. A. Gait says the Kāmarūpa mentioned in Yogini Tantra roughly included the Brahmaputra valley, Bhutan, Rangpur (in Bangladesh), Koch Bihar (in West Bengal), the North-East of Mymensing (in Bangladesh), and probably the Garo hills in Meghalaya.[15] This description is similar to what is mentioned in the Kālika Purāna as well. According to Kālika Purāna, the city of Pragjyotiṣpura is situated in the midst of Kāmarūpa, where the presiding deity is Kāmākhya. Upavīthī (branch-avenue), Vīthī (avenue), Upapīṭha, Pīṭha (holy site), Siddhapīṭha, Mahāpīṭha, Brahma-pīṭha, Visnupīṭha, Rudrapīṭha—these nine are called navayōni and situated in all the four directions of Kāmākhya. There is a region of 16 square kilometers, which is considered as the yōni maṇḍala, and in the midst of it exists manobhava-guhā, where Devī Kāmākhya resides in the red water (rakta pāniya rupini), which measures six square feet. According to Śrī Kālika Purāna, along with the worship of Kāmākhya, 64 Yoginis are to be worshipped.[16]

All of this points to one possibility—could it be that Ma Kāmākhya's abode is not just one temple in isolation, but the center of a sacred Śrī Cakra itself?[17]

Understanding Her through mantras

One of the ways in which we can understand who Ma Kāmākhya is is through her mantras, which are to be recited at various instances of the darśan. The mantras, rules, and rituals are given in Yogini Tantra. Some of those mantras are given below. The mantra by which she is to be invoked is as follows:

कामाख्ये कामसम्पन्ने कामेश्वरि हरप्रिये ।

कामनां देहि मे नित्यं कामेश्वरि नमोस्तुते ॥

kāmakhye kāmasampanne kāmeśvari harapriye

kāmanām dehi me nityam kāmeśvari namo stute

In the above mantra, she is hailed as Kāmeśvari, who satisfies all desires, and the devotee requests her to fulfill his desires every day.

Before visiting the sanctum, her salutation mantra is to be recited, as follows:

कामाख्ये वरदे देवी नीलपर्वतवासिनी ।

त्वं देवी जगतं मातर्योनिमुद्रे नमोस्तुते ॥

kāmakhye varade devī nīlaparvatavāsini

tvam devī jagatam mātaṛyōnimudre namo stute

This mantra recognizes Kāmākhya as the Devī who resides in the Nilachal hills. In the second line, she is invoked as the Universal Mother who is represented as the yōni.

Next, when the devotee reaches the yōni in the sanctum, the mantra to be recited is called the sparśa mantra, which has to be recited as one touches the yōni. This mantra offers important clues as to Ma Kāmākhya's true nature.

मनोभाव गुहमध्ये रक्तपानीय रूपिणी |

तस्य स्पर्षमात्रेण पुनर्जन्म न विद्यते ||

manobhava guhamadhye raktapāniya rupiṇi

tasyaḥ sparśamātreṇa punarjanma na vidyate

Here, she is recognized as the one residing in the cave in the form of the blood-colored water. By touching her yōni, we request her to break our cycle of birth and re-birth and grant us mukti.

The above mantra is the most significant clue as to who Ma Kāmākhya is. She is not just Kāli or Mahākāli; She is not just Tripurasundarī; She is not just Kameśvari; She is not only all the Daśa Mahā Vidyās put together, but rather the Source of all of her many manifestations. Kāmākhya is none other than Mahāmāyā.

Mahāmāyā is Śakti, the unmanifested form of Brahman, which is the cause of all the causes. When Brahman expressed the Will to see many forms of the One, it was made possible through Mahāmāya. She is the driving force behind creation. Without Her, everything will be static, like Śiva in his corpse-like form.

Śrī Kālika Purāna beautifully describes Mahāmāya as the one to whom the great Devas Brahma, Vishnu, and Śiva bow down, because She is the rajasik creative force in Brahma, the sattvik preservative force in Vishnu, and the tamasik destructive force in Rudra. Without Her, the Devas themselves will not be able to function.

The Devī Māhātmyam describes the many instances when the Devas, defeated by the asuras, invoked Mahāmāya to rescue them and bring back order in the world. In her battle against Sumbha and Nisumbha, the demon brothers, Mahāmāya brought forth from herself her various forms such as Kāli, Durga, Katyayini, Vaishnavi, Raudri, Brahmi, Narasimhi, and others, who took on the demons and slain every one of them. When Sumbha asks her to reveal who is helping her, she said, "I am alone and single in this world. Who is there other than Me here? See, all these many fighting with you are Myself. Now look at Me." As soon as Devī uttered these words, all those appearances of many entered into the body of Durga, and there was none but Devī, the Single.[18]

In Kāmākhya, she is not represented as a Devī with form and attributes, but rather as the Source of all the forms of Devī. How apt that she be represented as the yōni, the birth canal, through which the entire universe came into being. Going into the sanctum and coming in contact with the waters of her yōni will make us feel like we have finally reached home. Because home is where the womb is.

Of all her manifested forms, Devī Lalitha Tripurasundari (also referred to as Ṣoḍaśī), the presiding Devī of the sacred Śrī Cakra, is considered as her full manifestation, and hence she is often associated with Ma Kāmākhya. Devī Kamala (also called Lakṣmī) is the abode of aiśwarya or abundance, indicating the desire fulfilling aspects of Ma Kāmākhya. Devī Mātaṅgī (also called Saraswatī) is the one who leads devotees to Lalitha; she is the one who makes possible all creative manifestations and represents the aspects of knowledge and wisdom. These are the three forms of the mūrti that were kept outside the sanctum.

Kāmākhya for bhukti

In her manifestation as Kāmeśvari, she fulfills the desires of all devotees, since she is the Creatrix. She is the mother who fulfills the desires of her children. She does not have to be told what is needed. As all intuitive mothers, she just knows. It is said that all devotees experience the fulfillment of their desires after visiting Kāmākhya.

This is not just belief. Often, the things we pray for are aspects of our life that we are struggling with. When we understand cakras, we understand that our desires, emotions, and physical well-being are associated with specific cakras. Often, the things we desire and pray for have to do with a cakra which is not acting for us because it is not sufficiently energized. Since the Kāmākhya temple is capable of acting on all cakras, this temple makes it possible to take us to the next level of growth, materialistically and/or spiritually. It is not incorrect if each devotee describes his/her experience at Kāmākhya differently, and that's why there are so many names and versions of who she is. The caitanyam in this temple impacts each devotee differently, based on what they need.

For me, this place was really powerful in the viśuddhi cakra. This was exactly what I needed, as viśuddhi is the place of creative work. The energy and creativity to undertake literary and poetic work arise out of the viśuddhi cakra, when it is sufficiently energized. It is also the cakra which enables one to gain insights into the śāstras without instruction and gain knowledge of the ātman. If someone were to ask me how I have arrived at what I have written in this book, I can only attribute it to Her Grace.

Kāmākhya for mukti

What is the spiritual significance of Kāmākhya's menstruation?

Unlike the path of renunciation and letting go of desires associated with mokṣa dhams like Sabarimala, here the path is of fulfilling desires. The end objective is however the same – mukti. In order to attain mukti, one must be done with all desires and the karma associated with it. This can either be achieved by renunciation as we see in Sabarimala or by fulfillment of desires as we experience through Kāmākhya.

Whosoever comes in contact with Ma Kāmākhya will attain mukti, be it humans or animals. The human birth is considered essential to attain mukti. It is said that even the Devas will have to be born as humans in order to undertake the needed sādhana and finally merge with Brahman. So, when we see animals being sacrificed at her altar, it is to be understood that these animals will have a higher birth in the next life, bringing them closer to the possibility of mukti. That is why mantras are recited before the animal is sacrificed. The same happens for humans who come in contact with the waters of her yōni. But unlike animals who do not accumulate karma, we humans do. Before we are sacrificed at her altar for mukti, she will ensure that all our pending karma is completed by fulfilling our desires. It will be a mistake to think of her benevolence as an aspect that will help us live materialistically. As our mother, she knows better.

She will hold our hand and take us beyond, whether or not we are aware of it.

And this is where the spiritual significance of menstruation comes into being. The same yōni which is the birth canal through which life is born becomes the canal for the dissolution of life, at the time of menstruation. Menstruation is the process by which we break the cycle of birth and re-birth because it occurs as a result of life not being created. When Ma Kāmākhya menstruates, her power to dissolve creation is at its peak. It is for this reason that Tantriks and sādhus flock to Kāmākhya during her menstruation. This is the time when it becomes easy to attain mukti with minimal effort, simply by being in the presence of Ma Kāmākhya.

It is said that menstruating women tend to absorb the prāṇa of those around them when they menstruate. So, imagine what might be the impact of Ma Kāmākhya's power of absorption during her menstrual days. This is why her temple remains closed during those four days, as her power will be too much for mortal humans to bear.

In India, the spiritual understanding of menstruation is this: menstruation is the most effortless spiritual sādhana through which one can attain the ultimate goal of mukti. This is why menstruating women are both feared and revered. This profound understanding of the spiritual purpose of menstruation is why women who embody this possibility are revered, and menstruation itself is celebrated during Ambubachi.

References for Chapter 11

1. Māyā is often defined as Illusion. However, a more apt definition would be 'Experience in Time and Space of Self and Not-Self' as written by Sir John Woodroffe in his book Shakti and Shakta.
2. In Āyurved classics, yōni refers to the complete female reproductive system and individual organs independently. However, it is usually used to describe the vulva/female external genitals.
3. Rites and Rituals of Kamakhya, Kalika Purāṇa
4. Sati is an incarnation of Pārvathi, the wife of Śiva
5. A Tantrik is one who practices Tantra as a spiritual path
6. Described in my book 'Women & Sabarimala:Science behind Restrictions'. Notion Press, 2019
7. Dakṣiṇāyana - six months from the summer solstice to winter solstice
8. Trishul - the Trident weapon carried by Śiva, and often used to represent him
9. Note that not all temples associated with maṇipūra cakra have the same effect. For those pursuing the path of worldly life, maṇipūra cakra will have the effect of triggering ambition and drive to do well in materialistic aspects.
10. Makara is a legendary sea-creature in Hindu mythology.
11. Avalon, Arthur (Sir John Woodroffe). The Serpent Power: The Secrets of Tantric and Shaktic Yoga, 1919
12. Kamarupa Kingdom, Wikimedia Commons

13. Varanasi, also known as Banaras, is a city in Uttar Pradesh, which is a well-known pilgrim site in India.
14. Shastri, Biswanarayan. The Yogini Tantra. 1982
15. Sir Edward Albert Gait. A History of Assam, 1906
16. Śrī Kālika Purāṇa
17. Śrī Cakra is a complex geometry found in the Śrī Vidyā school of Hinduism, which is considered as a means to experience the Divine Feminine. It is said to be the abode of cosmic awareness. The center of this geometry, the bindu, a red dot, is said to be the origin of creation, merging back into which is the purpose of the upāsana. For more information, one can refer the book "Gifts from the Goddess" by Michael M. Bowden.
18. Swami Shivananada. The Devi Mahatamya. Chapter 10.
19. Bowden, Michael. M. Gifts from the Goddess: Dasa Mahavidyas, 45th Parallel Press, 2019.

CHAPTER 12

THE MYTH OF MENSTRUATION AS A RESULT OF INDRĀ'S SIN

A year ago, I received an email from a Sanyasini[1] associated with a well-known religious order in India. She had read some of my articles and was writing to ask my views on the famous mythological story of menstruation being a result of women incurring the guilt of Bhagvan Indrā's sin. She informed me that this is the story narrated by some religious leaders and writers to explain why menstruation makes women impure. This is definitely an incorrect interpretation.

The story

Śrīmad Bhāgavata Purāna (skanda 6, chapter 9) mentions the story of Indrā killing Vishvarūpa, who was the official paṇḍit of the Devās, and thereby incurring the sin of brāhma-hatya, that is, the sin of killing a brāhmaṇa, a learned man. Vishvarūpa was part human and part asura (demon) since his mother was an asura. As a result, he secretly offered one portion of his sacrifices for the well-being of the asuras. When Indrā, the ruler of Devās, heard about this, he took his bolt and smote off the three heads of Vishvarūpa. Thus, Indrā incurred the sin of brāhma-hatya. If Indrā desired, he could have freed himself from this sin, owing to his powers. Instead, he chose to accept the guilt and sin of murdering a brāhmaṇa. At the end of one year of penance, in order to cleanse himself of this sin, he approached the Earth, trees, women, and water to share one-fourth of his guilt and thereby free him from it. [2]

In return for accepting one-fourth of the sin, the Earth asked for the boon that whenever it is dug, the hollow created should be automatically filled up. The acceptance of Indrā's sin by the Earth is said to be the reason why some parts of the Earth are barren (such as the desert region). The trees asked for the boon that whenever the branches are chopped, it should be able to re-grow. Thus, the sap from trees is seen as the result of the trees accepting Indrā's sin. Water asked for the boon of increasing its volume when mixed with other liquids. Therefore, the presence of foam and bubbles on the surface of water is said to be the result of accepting a portion of Indrā's sin. When women were approached by Indrā, they asked for the boon of being able to enjoy the company of men at all times. The boon was granted. The indication among women for accepting one-fourth of Indrā's guilt is said to be the monthly menstruation.

Interpretations

Now, let us take a closer look at the phrases used with respect to women accepting one-fourth of Indrā's guilt, as mentioned in Śrīmad Bhāgavata Purāna. The same is given below:

शश्वत्कांमवरेणामहस्तुरियं जगृहु: स्त्रिय:।
रजोरुपेण तास्वमहो मासि मासि प्रदृश्यते ॥९॥

śaśvat-kāma-vareṇāṁhas turīyaṁ jagṛhuḥ striyaḥ
rajo-rūpeṇa tāsv aṁho māsi māsi pradṛśyate

śaśvat – perpetual; kāma – desires; vareṇāṁhas – because of the sin of; turīyaṁ - one-fourth; jagṛhuḥ - accepted; striyaḥ - women.

rajo-rūpeṇa – in the form of menstrual blood; tāsv – in them; aṁho – the sinful reaction; māsi māsi – monthly; pradṛśyate – is seen.

The above phrase has been interpreted in many ways, with one version[3] saying,

> "Women are as a class very lusty, and apparently their continuous lusty desires are never satisfied. In return for Bhagvwan Indrā's benediction that there would be no cessation to their lusty desires, women accepted one fourth of the sinful reactions for killing a brāhmaṇa. As a result of those reactions, women manifest the signs of menstruation every month."

Another writer[4] mentions that

> "One commits adharma, if he/she prevents the birth of a jivaatma, intentionally or unintentionally. This is so because, in many ways preventing a child from taking a birth is similar to murdering a person. The one-third of paapa (sin) of brahmahatya is incurred due to the failure of the egg to fertilize and become fit to host a jivaatma into the physical universe."

In another interpretation of this story, I heard a man refer to menstruation as a great sacrifice by women because they accepted the sin of Indrā! Menstruation can only be a sacrifice if women are losing something in the process. But it is exactly the opposite. Besides, why would Indrā punish women for doing him a favor and taking his sin?

I have no doubt that these men mean well and are trying hard to give answers about a topic they can't possibly know enough about. Their attempts remind me of a beautiful quote by Swami Vivekananda when someone urged him to do something for the welfare of women. Swamiji said:

"Women will work out their destinies — much better, too, than men can ever do for them. All the mischief to women has come because men undertook to shape the destiny of women."

The real meaning of Indrā's story

The time has come to set the record straight and narrate this story as it is meant to be understood. Stories from the Purāṇas are beautifully told with the purpose of conveying deep philosophical ideas through simple tales. As with most ancient Hindu texts, the true meaning is often coded and hidden in the outwardly simplistic narration. Therefore, these stories are not to be taken literally and translated word-to-word. One has to understand the underlying message in such stories.

All stories in the Purāṇas have one basic goal—to shift the reader toward a spiritual outlook with the understanding that mukti is the ultimate reason for birth as a human. In order to attain mukti, it is necessary for humans to break the karmic cycle of birth and re-birth. Until we are able to do that, it is believed that we will be born again and again. So, how can a spiritual aspirant break the cycle of birth and re-birth?

One of the essential aspects of the spiritual path is to be able to withhold the human seed, contained in semen in men and menstrual blood in women. The seed is then transformed into subtler forms by making it rise higher up the cakras, through certain practices under the guidance of a Guru. This process is known to practitioners of Tantra as well as Taoism.

In this pursuit of mukti, there will be a conflict if one engages in sexual activities that involve the release of the human seed. That is why advanced tantric techniques teach how to engage in sexual activity without releasing the seed/semen. In the absence of this knowledge, for men pursuing intense spiritual sādhana, it is a necessity to preserve the semen through the practice of celibacy. By observing celibacy, men consciously choose to break the cycle of birth and re-birth. But for women, celibacy is not necessary, since menstruation is the process by which women break the karma of birth and re-birth. If menstruation is brāhma-hatya, then celibacy practiced by men is too. In fact, more so, because unlike menstruation, which is involuntary, celibacy is a voluntary choice to not bring forth life. But while the latter is considered as a high spiritual path, menstruation is considered as a sin. How can we have such contradictory ideas?

There is a line in Vasiṣṭha Dharmasūtra which says, "For month on month the menstrual excretion takes away her sins." Unlike the black and white notion of good and bad considered as sin in many religions, in the Hindu religion, anything that takes us away from achieving the goal of mukti is considered a sin. In this story of Indrā, by 'sin', it is meant the karma of creating life and all the attachments it brings which make the process of mukti that much more difficult. Therefore, the 'boon' that women received from Indrā, in return for the favor of taking away one-fourth of his sin, is the ability to pursue the spiritual path without having to follow celibacy. Menstruation is the process that makes this possible. This essentially means that women can enjoy a marital/sexual life and, at the same time, follow a spiritual path. In other words, both bhukti and mukti are attainable through a female body. This is made possible through the natural phases of menstruation and menopause.

Spirituality for women

For men, celibacy is practiced in the form of Brahmacārya, which encompasses a number of spiritual practices besides sexual abstinence. Men who are on such a path will be able to transform the human seed into subtler forms that power their personality and spiritual capacity. In Āyurved, the seventh tissue layer or dhātu is called śukra dhātu. This is the last dhātu; the food that we ingest will become subtler and go into the formation of this layer which constitutes the reproductive essence of ovum in women and semen in men. For common people, this layer is depleted through sexual activity. For one practicing Brahmacārya, the śukra becomes transformed into ojas, which enhances the cellular immunity, and tejas, the mental fire to achieve whatever one sets one's mind to.

This possibility is naturally available to women once they enter the realm of menopause. That is why, in India, menopause is closely associated with spirituality since a woman's body will now be able to experience spiritual heights without it interfering with menstrual and reproductive processes. Often, we think that because women menstruate, they are not able to pursue a spiritual path like men. The truth is that women do not have to do all the sādhana that men do as long as they menstruate. The legendary stories of women like Meerabai and Akkamahadevi, my own experiences, and that of other women like me, who are neither initiated nor undertake intense sādhana like a Yogin and yet are able to perceive subtler aspects easily, are testimony to what menstruation can do for women. While menstruation offers women the chance to experience and enjoy life while tuning their body to experience the subtler realm more easily, menopause offers the possibility of spiritual enlightenment. Therefore, nature has created women in such a way that her body and her mind will naturally lead her to fulfill her karma and also attain mukti, with the least effort. This is the boon granted by Indrā to women, in return for accepting one-fourth of his sin.

Meaning of rajaswala

Some men have wrongly interpreted rajaswala, the term for menstruating women, as a time when women are full of rajas, that is, a time for activity and action.[4] But women who menstruate know by experience that what they feel is a state of non-action. The more apt interpretation would be that rajaswala is one in whom the quality of rajas[5] is flowing out. When rajas, the quality of action, is leaving a woman's body, she becomes either full of sattva, the quality of harmony and purity, or is overcome with tamas, the quality of inertia and laziness, based on her disposition. By nature, most women are rajasic and tend to tilt toward an action-oriented lifestyle. But once a month, all women feel the natural urge to stay still when menstruation occurs. This is the leaving of rajas – rajaswala.

Yōg sūtras[6] provide insights into how the mind functions when influenced by the three guṇas of sattva, rajas, and tamas. Sattva is the quality of illumination; rajas is the quality of action; tamas is the quality of inertia. When the mental essence manifesting as sattva is mixed with rajas and tamas, then the love for power and sense objects occurs. The same under the influence of tamas approaches vice, ignorance, desire, and laziness. When the same has overcome the veil of illusion and has a touch of rajas, then we see virtue, knowledge, mastery, and desirelessness. When even the touch of rajas is removed, then it shows forth the distinction between prakṛti (matter) and puruṣa (consciousness) and approaches a state of trance called dharma-megha (cloud of virtue). This, the thinkers call the highest intellection – param prasaṅkhyānam.

It is within every woman's capacity to recognize the opportunity that menstruation brings and tap into it for a higher purpose. It is the time when women turn inward, effortlessly. Menstruation, in itself, can be a spiritual sādhana. For one who understands this, menstruation is not a hurdle; it is the path itself.

References for Chapter 12

1. A woman ascetic who has taken the path of renunciation
2. This story also features in other texts such as Taittirīya Saṃhita, Vasiṣṭha Dharmasūtra and Garuḍa Purāṇa, with some modifications
3. https://prabhupadabooks.com/sb/6/9/9
4. Sridhar, Nithin. The Sabarimala Confusion - Menstruation Across Cultures. 2019
5. This is a reference to the three gunas of Sattva, Rajas and Tamas
6. Prasada, Rama. The Sacred Book of the Hindus, The Yōga Sutras of Patanjali, Vol IV, 1924

CHAPTER 13

MENSTRUAL PRACTICES IN CHRISTIANITY AND ISLAM

At the introduction of this book, there is an overview of the similarity of ancient sciences across the world. The cultural and religious practices of a region are often influenced by their knowledge of native science. So, naturally, the question arises about menstrual regulations in other religions. Do Christian women follow menstrual restrictions? What about Muslim women? And why do Sikh women not have any menstrual regulations? This chapter will attempt to answer these questions.

Understanding the depth of any one religion should make it possible for us to understand other religions and their practices to a certain extent. We might even be surprised to find the similarities that exist at the core of religions that seem to be at loggerheads on the surface. Over the years, as I explored menstrual practices associated with different religious groups, I found that at the core, these practices were rooted in the understanding of subtle sciences. It seems as though our ancestors across the world were far too familiar with the subtleties of how the human body functions and evolved practices around this understanding. Their familiarity was such that they perhaps thought it was unnecessary to explain the 'why' behind practices, especially menstrual practices, as it must have seemed obvious to them.

Ancient religions and the practices they evolved have layers of understanding—the ritualistic layer, the symbolic layer, the faith-based layers—and underneath it all lies the scientific layer, from which the rest seemed to have been created. As we explore the various menstrual practices across different religious communities, this similarity in scientific knowledge of ancient religions becomes more and more evident.

Menstrual regulations among Christian women

> "And if a woman have an issue, [and] her issue in her flesh be blood, she shall be put apart seven days: and whosoever toucheth her shall be unclean until the even. And every thing that she lieth upon in her separation shall be unclean: every thing also that she sitteth upon shall be unclean. And whosoever toucheth her bed shall wash his clothes, and bathe [himself] in water, and be unclean until the even. And whosoever toucheth any thing that she sat upon shall wash his clothes, and bathe [himself] in water, and be unclean until the even. And if it [be] on [her] bed, or on any thing whereon she sitteth, when he toucheth it, he shall be unclean until the even. And if any man lie with her at all, and her flowers be upon him, he shall be unclean seven days; and all the bed whereon he lieth shall be unclean."
>
> – Leviticus, Chapter 15, (19-24), King James' Bible

The regulations on menstruating women and women who have given birth to a child (Lev 12. 1-5) are mentioned in the Old Testament Book of Leviticus in the Bible. While menstruating women were considered unclean for the duration of their menstrual flow, women who had just given birth were also considered unclean and kept in seclusion for a period of 40 days. These practices are very similar to what Hindu women have been following even today. However, most Christian women are unaware of the existence of these rules in the Old Testament.

I first encountered menstrual practices among Christian women during one of our field visits in a village in the Uttara Kannada district of Karnataka. The Christian women who were interviewed said that while it is okay for menstruating women in their community to visit the church, the priest had told them to refrain from receiving the Holy Communion during menstruation. I later learned that among Orthodox Christians, it is widely practiced that menstruating women refrain from receiving the Holy Communion (consecrated bread and wine which is considered as the body and blood of Christ). The consecration of bread and wine into the body and blood of Christ is known as the Holy Eucharist.

Unlike a Hindu temple, the building of a church is not what is consecrated. Instead, it is through the celebration of the Holy Eucharist that the spiritual possibility is made accessible to individuals. In fact, even the language used during the ritual is Syriac/Syrian, which is said to be derived from Aramaic. Aramaic is the language that Jesus is believed to have spoken. The primal sounds of ancient languages were known to invoke subtler forces that could impact the physical body. Just as Saṃskṛtam verses produce sound vibrations that can alter the biological forces in the human body, the Syrian language too must have had a similar effect and hence it was used while consecrating the bread and wine. In South India's Orthodox churches, we find that the ancient Syrian language, called Suryani[1] in Kerala, is still used during the Holy Eucharist, even though the rest of the sermon is in an Indian language. Therefore, the portion of the Christian ritual which is likely to impact the subtle bodily forces is the Holy Eucharist, not the church itself. In this light, the regulation on menstruating women from accepting the Holy Communion can be understood.

It should be noted that most Catholic and Protestant churches in India have translated the entire sermon, including the sacred recitation during the Holy Eucharist, into Indian languages. The intention here was to make a foreign religion relatable to the natives of a new region. However, in the process of Indianizing the church, the sacred aspects of consecration have been lost. Whereas the Orthodox church and other sects of Christianity that follow the Old Testament have continued to safeguard the ancient language and customs to a large extent, and hence we see the menstrual regulation among those practicing the Orthodox Christian religion.

Menstrual regulations among Muslim women

For Muslim women, religion-based menstrual regulations require them to not perform the Namaz/Salat or read the Quran during menstruation. They are also restricted from fasting on Ramadan during menstruation.

Those who are familiar with Yōg āsanas will recognize the postures taken during Namaz to include semi-paschimottāsana (ruku pose), shashankāsana (sujud pose), and vajrāsana (julus pose). Each of the five prayer positions has a corresponding yōga position.[2]

Paschimottāsana and shashankāsana direct the flow of blood toward the upper body parts and higher cakras, which could reverse the apāna vāyu during menstruation. Vajrāsana activates the samāna and apāna vāyu, thereby regulating digestion and movement of wastes out of the body. However, for menstruating women, the apāna vāyu is already active and when further stimulated, especially five times as it is supposed to be repeated during Namaz every day, it could increase the menstrual flow. Hence, these āsanas or rather Namaz is restricted for menstruating women.

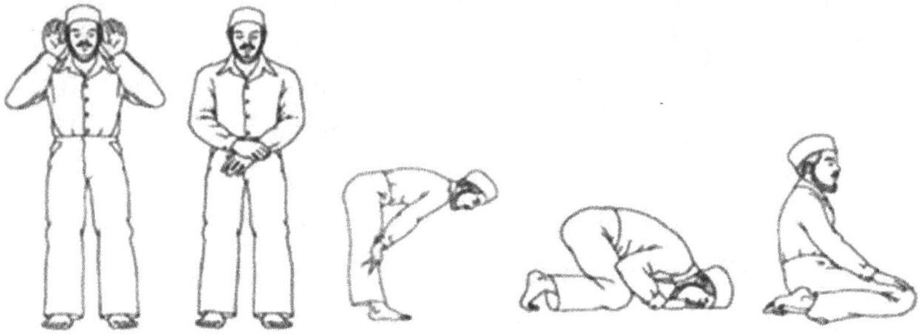

Figure 21: The different postures during Namaz

Image Source: http://www.islam-hinduism.com/hindu-yoga-and-the-five-prayers-in-islam-23/

Like Saṃskṛtam and Syrian, the Quran's language is Arabic. Arabic is also an ancient language which produces the sound vibrations capable of impacting the subtle forces by activating the cakras. Virtually all of the sounds of the Arabic language are uttered while reciting Quran, creating a balance in all affected areas of the body. During Ramadan, Muslims are required to fast and read the Quran. Activation of the cakras is most effective when done on an empty stomach, and the same is recommended even in Hinduism. However, this is not prescribed for menstruating women as it will impact menstruation.

Why the Gurudwara has no menstrual regulation

When we closely look at menstrual practices across different religions, we find that menstrual restrictions are imposed on entering spaces that are ritually consecrated or on partaking in rituals that cause the apāna vāyu to change its direction by activating higher cakras. In order to understand the absence of menstrual restrictions in religions such as Sikhism, the questions to be explored are:

- Whether or not the religious space is ritually consecrated (not just symbolically)?
- Do they follow rituals involving ancient languages or poses similar to yōga āsanas?

Exploring these questions with respect to a Gurudwara should lead us to the answers we are looking for. Sikhism evolved as a reformist movement and is one of the youngest religions. At its core, it strove to move away from ritualistic practices and convey the essence of religion in the common language of the masses. The focus here is not on consecrated spaces or primal sounds, and therefore, the lack of menstrual regulations in a Gurudwara is obvious.

Lastly, when we explore religion and science in an unbiased fashion, we will realize that ancient religions have more in common than what we like to admit. The impact of a Hindu temple on a menstruating woman is similar to receiving the Holy Communion for an Orthodox Christian woman or performing the Namaz/Salat for a Muslim woman. Religion was considered as an effective tool to imbibe scientific understanding among the masses, and rituals/religious practices evolved in this background. Has it been misused? Perhaps yes. But calling all of it as superstition is actually a new level of superstition, since it comes without the curiosity and exploration that religion might have wanted us to cultivate.

References for Chapter 13

1. Basheer, K.P.M. Suriyani: A sacred language is vanishing from the State. The Hindu. 11-Aug-2008
2. https://archive.islamonline.net/797

NOTES

1

DARŚANA

Out of the six systems of Indian philosophy (Darśana), Āyurved is said to have been influenced by the Sāṃkhya, Yōg, Nyāya and Vaiśeṣika philosophies. Information about these systems of philosophy is given below in some detail. The reference for the below text is largely from the series of publications by various Saṃskṛtam scholars under the title "The Sacred Book of Hindus."

I. Sāṃkhya Darśana by ācārya Kapila

Sāṃkhya philosophy explains the Theory of Causation (parināmvād) as the coming together of puruṣa (pure consciousness) and prakṛti (inert matter) with the infusion of 25 tatvas. By Tatva is meant the Tva, i.e., condition or existence of Tat, or that by which all the three worlds are pervaded. Sāṃkhya mentions these 25 tatvas as:

1. Prakṛti (unmanifest material cause/matter)
2. Buddhi (cosmic intelligence), also referred to as Mahat
3. Ahaṃkāra (Self-assertion or ego or the 'I' factor)
4. Five tanmātras (perception): gandha – smell, rasa – taste, rūpa – form, sparśa – touch, śabda – sound/hearing

5. Five Mahābhūtas (5 elements): pṛthvi – earth, āpās or jal – water, agni – fire, vāyu – air, ākāśa – ether
6. Five Jñānendriyas (Sense organs): ghrāṇa – nose, jihva – tongue, cakṣu – eye, tvak – skin, śrotra – ear
7. Five Karmendriyas (5 motor faculties): pāyu - the excretory organ, upastha - the sexual organs, pāda - the locomotion organ/legs, pāni - the organ of apprehension/ hands, vāk - the speech organ
8. Manas (Mind)
9. Apart from the above 24 tatvas, there is puruṣa, the 25th tatva, which is the realm of Pure Consciousness, or Knower, and is considered as separate from the above.

Due to the recognition of two factors, viz., puruṣa and prakṛti, sāṃkhya philosophy is also called Dualistic Realism.

Sāṃkhya also lays down three pramāṇas (proof of knowledge) as reliable methods to arrive at the correct knowledge. These methods are pratyakṣa (perception), anumāna (inference), āptavacana (testimony from a reliable source). An interesting aspect which sāṃkhya propounds is the idea of emergence of truth by ruling out the untruth - na iti na iti, which means, 'not this, not this'. To give a familiar example, when Sir Thomas Edison said "I have not failed. I've just found 10,000 ways that won't work", it can be said to be the application of Sāṃkhya philosophy. Spiritual Liberation, too, is defined in this way as the absence of suffering, rather than the presence of enjoyment.

Sāṃkhya's theory of causation with 25 tatvas is important, as it is accepted and applied in Vedānta as well as in Tantra, and is considered as understood in Āyurved. The three pramāṇas find mention in Caraka Saṃhitā as scientific methods for obtaining facts about the patient being treated. In addition, Caraka added yukti, meaning rationale or common sense, as the fourth pramāṇa. Further, the role of buddhi, ahaṃkāra and manas described in Sāṃkhya as creating mental modifications causing pain or pleasure is recognized in Āyurved by the way in which mental health is considered as an integral part of overall wellbeing. Consequently, Deha-Mānasa (psychosomatic) approach is an important contribution of Caraka Saṃhitā in the field of medicine.

Triguṇa

Sāṃkhya also proposes the theory of the three guṇa (qualities) of prakṛti namely, Sattva, Rajas and Tamas, the interplay of which begins the process of creation. In a simplified manner, Sattva, the Essence, is said to be light and illuminating, Rajas, the Energy, is said to be exciting and restless, while Tamas, the Mass, is said to be heavy and dull. Prakṛti contains within it the three guṇas and it is non-intelligent, i.e. it does not act on its own. Puruṣa, on the other hand, does not contain the guṇas (a state of no qualities) and is the intelligent knower, observer and experiencer, but it is a non-agent. Therefore, according to Sāṃkhya, it is the coming together of puruṣa and prakṛti that results in creation.[1]

The guṇas (Reals), though assuming an infinite diversity of forms and powers, can neither be created nor destroyed. The totality of the Mass (Tamas), as well as of Energy (Rajas), remains constant, if we take account both of the manifested and the unmanifested, the actual and the potential. But the individual products of the evolutionary process resulting from the combined action of the original Mass (Tamas), Energy (Rajas), and Essence (Sattva) are subject to addition and subtraction, growth and decay, resulting in a continuous process of creation.

Buddhi, Ahaṃkāra & Manas

Buddhi springs from prakṛti and in its turn, gives rise to ahaṃkāra; ahaṃkāra, in its turn, gives rise to the tanmātras of sound, touch, smell, form, and taste; and these, in their turn, gives rise respectively to the elements of ether, air, earth, fire, and water. And finally, the gross indriya (sense and motor organs) and mind.

When a human perceives something with his indriya, it is the manas which considers, ahaṃkāra which identifies and buddhi which determines the course of action. The action of these can be instantaneous or successive, as described below:

- Instantaneous – Ex: When one suddenly comes across a tiger in a dark night, one's eyes at once observe, manas considers, ahaṃkāra identifies, and buddhi determines course of action and the man immediately runs away for his life.
- Successive – Ex: when a man sees in dim light something moving in front of him and doubt arises as to what it might be, his manas considers that it is nothing but a robber; his ahaṃkāra makes him self-conscious that the robber is approaching towards him; and his buddhi determines that he must move away.

In Sāṃkhya, it is established that buddhi is supreme among the indriyas. It is the principal means of accomplishing the apparently contradictory purposes of puruṣa, viz., experience and release. Buddhi fulfils puruṣa's desire to experience, for experience consists in the apprehension of pleasure and pain, and this exists in buddhi. And while, on the one hand, it is the cause of experience, it is, on the other hand, the cause of release as well, since it is through buddhi that one can cause discrimination between prakṛti and puruṣa, leading to release of puruṣa from the bondage of experience.

Five vital airs

Sāṃkhya also talks of the five vital airs, viz., prāṇa, udāna, vyāna, samāna and apāna, that arise out of the modifications of the buddhi, ahaṃkāra and manas (and not of the elements).

Sāṃkhya's idea of liberation

The core of Sāṃkhya philosophy is interesting in that it teaches one to go beyond karma and not to waste one's time on rituals, etc. that are supposed to help one break free from karma. Sāṃkhya says that to attain liberation, there is no need for atonement and redemption (from karma) or even to lead the life of an ascetic. Instead, Sāṃkhya teaches that if one were to acquire the ability of distinguishing or discriminating the unmanifest prakṛti, the manifest tatvas and the knower puruṣa, then that alone will lead to liberation. This discriminating ability is called viveka or vijñāna, which when acquired will automatically free one of all karmic bonds. Enlightenment is described as the state where one is free of all suffering and pain, as pain is not a condition of the Pure Self.

Karma is distinguished as prārabdha or operative (gathered during the course of current life), sañcita or accumulated (impressions from previous births), and āgamika, or to come, or future. On the attainment of discriminative knowledge (viveka), sañcita karma or karma in seed-form is burnt up and rendered infructuous, and āgamika karma also is necessarily precluded. Only the prārabdha then remains, which needs to be worked out by the body before its end. When discriminative knowledge is perfectly developed before the prārabdha has worked itself out, the incarnate puruṣa is released, but remains awhile burdened with the body. This is what is called Jivan-Mukti or the state of release/liberation during life. When (in due course) separation from the body takes place, and there is cessation of the activity of the prakṛti from her purpose having been fulfilled, puruṣa attains both absolute and final Kaivalya. However, Sāṃkhya philosophy is clear that such thinking has to be applied to the higher Self in the pursuit of spiritual liberation, and not in day-to-day life.

Sāṃkhya philosophy does not talk of a God as a typical creator, although later schools of Sāṃkhya has included it. Regarding cause and effect, Sāṃkhya's take is that the effect is pre-existent in the cause, because that which is non-existent, can by no means be brought into existence.

Source:

- Lecture on Sāṃkhya Philosophy by Swami Samarpananada, Indian Spiritual Heritage
- Sinha, Nandalal. The Sacred Book of the Hindus, Sāṃkhya Philosophy Vol X1, 1915
- Seal, Brajendranath. The Positive Sciences of the Ancient Hindus, 1915

II. Yōg Sūtras by ācārya Patanjali

Sāṃkhya and Yōg have the same metaphysics, which speaks of creation resulting from the coming together of puruṣa (consciousness) and prakṛti (inert matter). But the difference lies in the approach towards spiritual realization. While Sāṃkhya deals with the theoretical knowledge, Yōg provides practical methods of realization.

Sūtra means an aphorism. The aphorisms of Patanjali on Yōg are nearly 200 in number. The word Yōg comes from Saṃskṛtam root which means 'to go to trance or to meditate'. Others, however derive it from a root which means union or to join. The philosophy of Patanjali is essentially dualistic, with three eternal co-existent principles of puruṣa, prakṛti and Īśvara (God).

Yōg is defined as citta-vṛtti-nirodhah, i.e. restraining the vṛtti (reaction) of the citta (mind). In other words, Yōg is the restraint of mental modifications. The thought-vehicle (manas), the I-vehicle (ahaṃkāra) and the pure-reason-vehicle (buddhi) constitute citta or the subtlest form of matter. To free man from the fetters of this citta is the purpose of Yōg. When the mind has become fully restrained, there is the realization that man is not the body nor the mind; instead he is Pure Consciousness (puruṣa). In this stage, man is said to be in his original form or Svarūpa.

Classification of the mind

Yōg describes 5 different types of mind as seen in human beings.

1. Kṣipta - Hyperactive or wandering mind, which takes in pleasure and pain

2. Mūḍha - Forgetful, Self-centered or dull mind, which tends to injure others for their self-interest
3. Vikṣipta - Occasionally steady or distracted mind
4. Ekāgra - one pointed, highly concentrated mind. Such a mind can focus and concentrate on any subject
5. Niruddha - Restrained mind where cessation of reactions and thoughts occur, that is, complete stopping of mind. In this state, there will be spiritual realization.

Classification of vṛtti

The first four types of minds are always active, moving and creating mental waves, resulting in five kinds of vṛtti:

1. Pramāṇa - objective reality that is understood through senses (pratyakṣa), inference (anumāna) and scriptures (āptavacana)
2. Viparyāya - unreal cognition or illusion
3. Vikalpa - Imagination, hallucination or verbal delusion
4. Nidrā - Deep sleep or non-perception of anything external
5. Smṛityaḥ - Memory or reviving of old perception

These vṛttis create intellectual and emotional modifications of the citta. The intellectual aspect is to be controlled by abhyāsa, that is, by training the mind to focus on one object. The emotional aspect has to be checked by practice of vairāgya or detachment from worldly emotions of pain or pleasure, attraction or repulsion, love or hatred, etc.

Afflictions

Yōg also talks about the afflictions, both intellectual and emotional, which affect every human being. These are:

1. Avidyā - nescience or wrong notion of things objective, such as mistaking the non-eternal for the eternal, the impure for the pure, the painful for the pleasurable, the non-self for the self, and so on.
2. Asmitā - wrong notion of things subjective, such as identifying one's Self (ātman) with the vehicle in which the Self functions (body)
3. Rāga - the natural desire of man, running after pleasant things
4. Dveṣa - hatred of things that give pain
5. Abhiniveśa - the instinct of self-preservation

Yōg says that these afflictions are the root cause of birth, re-birth and suffering, and can be overcome by meditation.

Disturbances of the mind

The Yōg Sūtras classify the disturbances of the mind into 9 categories:

1. vyādhi (disease) - disturbance of the equilibrium of the humours, chyle and the organs of the body
2. styāna (languor) - indisposition of the mind to work
3. saṃśaya (indecision) - notion touching both sides of the question: it may or it may not be
4. pramāda (carelessness) -the want of resort to the means of trance
5. ālasya (sloth) - inertia of mind and body consequent upon heaviness
6. avirati (sensuality) - the desire consequent of objects of sense having taken possession of the mind

7. bhrānti – mistaken notion which is false knowledge
8. darśana-alabdha-bhumikatva – missing the point, this is the non-attainment of the state of trance
9. anavasthithatva (instability) – incapacity of the mind to keep in any state that has been attained, because it becomes stable only when the state of trance has been reached

These distractions of the mind are said to be the enemies and obstacles of Yōg. The Yōg Sūtras provide important insights into how the mind functions, the disturbances which affect the mind and how to gain mastery over the mind. The Yōg Sūtras recognize vyādhi or disease as a disturbance of the mind, and this understanding can be seen incorporated into Āyurved, especially in its understanding of disease prevention. Unlike in modern medicine which has compartmentalized mental health as separate from physical health, Āyurved has always understood the connection between the two.

Aṣṭāṅga Yōg

Every impulse has a meaning associated with it and there is a knowledge about it – śabda (sound), artha (meaning), jñāna (knowledge) – these three are connected inextricably. A Yōgi has to be in such control of the mind that he can separate/distinguish these three stages and control his reactions (vṛtti). To do this, there are eight steps:

1. Yama – Practice of restraint by controlling basic impulses. This includes ahimsa (abstinence from injury), satya (veracity), asteya (abstinence from theft), brahmacārya (continence & celibacy), aparigraha (abstinence from avariciousness)

2. Niyama - Observance or practice of certain virtues such as śauca (cleanliness in body and mind), santoṣa (contentment), tapah (asceticism and austerity), svādhyāya (study of sacred books), īśvara - pranidhānani (making īśvara the motive of all actions)
3. Āsana - Postures that can be maintained in a steady and easy way without inducing pain
4. Prāṇayāma - Regulation of breath
5. Pratyāhāra - Pratyāhāra is that by which the senses do not come into contact with their objects, and as it were, follow the nature of the mind. The senses are restrained, like the mind, when the mind is restrained. It is a stage of catalepsy where the senses do not come into contact with their objects.
6. Dhāraṇā - Concentration or to focus the mind. When the Yōgi reaches catalepsy, he fixes his mind on any particular portion of his body. This holding of the mind in a particular part is called dhāraṇā.
7. Dhyān – Meditation. The continuation of the Yōgi's effort to keep the mind focussed in dhāraṇā is dhyān.
8. Samādhi – The cessation of activities of the mind. Dhyān turns into samādhi when the sense of self is lost and only the object of meditation remains in the mind.

While the first five are external practices or bahiraṅga, the last three are internal practices or antaraṅga yōg. When dhāraṇā, dhyān and samādhi are performed together, it is called saṃyama, which is considered to be the method of acquiring all knowledge of super-sensuous verities. It is the great light of wisdom called prajñaloka. For one who has mastered saṃyama, various siddhis (psychic powers) will manifest, such as knowledge of past, present and future, reading thoughts of others, disappearance from sight, seeing through closed doors, knowledge of the solar system and astronomy, etc. These methods can only be comprehended by one who has experienced saṃyama.

For example, it is said that by practicing saṃyama on the navel, one will gain knowledge of the human system. The knowledge of the doṣas (vital humor), dhātu (tissue), nāḍī (subtle channel), and subtle human anatomy expounded in Āyurved could have been gained through this method, by one who has mastered saṃyama. This would also explain why the scientists and physicians of ancient India were often seers who had mastered such techniques and hence could access higher faculties of knowledge. Using a similar technique, Dr. Annie Besant and C.W. Leadbeater gained unique insights into the structure of chemical elements and published their findings in the book Occult Chemistry. What Indian sages called saṃyama, the theosophists called clairvoyance.

Source:

- ✦ Lecture on Yōg Sūtras by Swami Samarpananada, Indian Spiritual Heritage
- ✦ Prasada, Rama. The Sacred Book of the Hindus, The Yōg Sūtras of Patanjali, Vol IV, 1924

III. Nyāya Darśana by ācārya Gautama

Nyāya means logic. Nyāya darśana expounded by ācārya Gautama is considered as the school of Logical Realism, with its fine understanding of the science of reasoning (tarka śāstra). Nyāya darśana believes in obtaining knowledge by proofs (pramāṇa) & critical logic. Nyāya philosophy is bold in the way it dismisses all methods of arriving at the truth, which are not scientific, logical and can be reasoned.

The methods of Nyāya Sūtras, like that of Vaiśeṣika, consists in the enumeration, definition and examination of categories. The Nyāya Sūtras treats of four distinct subjects:

1. tarka - The art of debate
2. pramāṇa - The means of valid knowledge
3. avayava - The doctrine of syllogism
4. anyamata-parīkṣā - The examination of contemporaneous philosophical doctrines

The first two subjects combined together form the tarka śāstra (the philosophy of reasoning). Nyāya describes the four sources of knowledge as pratyakṣa (direct perception), anumāna (inference), upamāna (analogy/comparison), śabda (verbal testimony).

1. pratyakṣa or perception, is defined as that knowledge which arises from the contact of a sense with its objects, and which is determinate, unnamable and non-erratic.
2. anumāna or inference, is knowledge which is preceded by perception and is of three kinds, viz., a priori (knowledge of effect from perception of cause), a

posteriori (knowledge of cause from perception of its effect) and commonly seen (knowledge of one thing derived from the perception of another thing with which it is commonly seen)

3. upamāna or comparison, is knowledge of a thing through its similarity to another thing previously known
4. śabda or verbal testimony refers to the knowledge gained from the instructive assertion of a reliable person.

These four methods of nyāya based on the physical experience of things, have been made use of extensively in the study of action of various drugs included in Indian medicine. Thus, the contribution of the nyāya system of philosophy to Āyurved in establishing scientific methodology is very important.

Nyāya says that supreme felicity is attained by the knowledge of the true nature of 16 categories. Knowledge about the true nature of the 16 categories mentioned below means true knowledge by the enunciation, definition and critical examination of the categories. The 16 categories are:

1. pramāṇa – means of right knowledge
2. prameya – object of right knowledge
3. saṃśaya – doubt; which is a conflicting judgement about the precise character of an object, arising from the recognition of properties common to many objects, or of properties not common to any object, from conflicting testimony, and from irregularity of perception and non-perception
4. prayojana – purpose; purpose is that with an eye to which one proceeds to act

5. dṛṣṭāntata – familiar instance; a familiar instance is a thing about which an ordinary man and an expert entertain the same opinion
6. siddhānta – established tenet; an established tenet is a dogma resting on the authority of a certain school, hypothesis or implication
7. avayava – doctrine of syllogism, which includes proposition, reason, example, application and conclusion
8. tarka – debate, confutation; confutation is carried on for ascertaining the real character of a thing of which the character is not known. It is reasoning which reveals the character by showing the absurdity of all contrary characters.
9. nirṇaya – ascertainment; refers to the removal of doubt, and the determination of a question, by hearing two opposite sides
10. vāda – discussion
11. jalpah – sophistry, wrangling; a wrangler is one who, engaged in a disputation, aims only at victory, being indifferent whether his arguments support his own contention or that of the opponent, provided he can make out a pretext for bragging that he has taken an active part in the debate
12. vitaṇḍā – cavil; a caviller does not endeavour to establish anything, but confines himself to mere carping at the arguments of his opponents
13. hetvabhāsa – fallacy; fallacies of a reason are the erratic, the contradictory, the equal to the question, the unproved, and the mistimed

14. chalam - quibble; quibble is the opposition offered to a proposition by the assumption of an alternative meaning. It is of three kinds - quibble in respect of a term, of a genus or of a metaphor

15. jātih - futility; futility consists in offering objections founded on mere similarity or dissimilarity

16. nigrahasthānam - occasion for rebuke; an occasion for rebuke arises when one misunderstands or does not understand at all

Nyāya also acknowledges the pañca mahābhūtas (earth, fire, air, water, ether) and the sensations associated with each of these such as touch, smell, etc. Nyāya spoke of atoms as being the thing of the smallest dimension; two atoms form a dvyaṇuka (dyad) and three dvyaṇukas make a tryasarenu (triad). All things which can be perceived are composed of triads. This is similar to what is mentioned in the Vaiśeṣika and forms the basis of Āyurved's tridoṣa system.

Nyāya differs from other darśanas in its understanding of the soul (ātman) as a substance that feels pain, pleasure, desire, etc. Here, soul is said to be not self-conscious until it comes in contact with the mind & senses. Liberation, therefore is to disjoint the soul from the mind & senses.

Nyāyaiks said that Reality is that which is knowable and namable by language (opposite of Vedānta which says that true reality cannot be known by language and cannot be named). Nyāyaiks said that it is not the limitation of language, rather the human incapacity of knowing reality which is the real limitation. And therefore, they created this logical reasoning language.

According to Nyāya, there are three types of false persuasions – false persuasion by speech, by generalization and by figure. There is also false persuasion by universality, that is, agreeing to something because it is universally agreed to by many. Nyāya says that giving up one's perseverance because of a rigid belief may lead to uncertainty. But a contemplative investigation of that very uncertainty may lead to spiritual liberation. Thus, Nyāya encourages individuals to pursue the truth on their own through deep contemplation and reasoning, rather than take someone else's word as true.

Source:

1. Vidyabhusana, Satish Chandra. The Sacred Book of the Hindus, The Nyaya Sutras of Gotama, Vol VIII, 1930
2. Keith, A.B. Indian Logic and Atomism: An exposition of the Nyaya and Vaiśeṣika systems, 1921
3. Lecture on Nyāya Philosophy by Swami Samarpananda, Indian Spiritual Heritage

IV. Vaiśeṣika darśana by ācārya Kanada

Vaiśeṣika darśana by ācārya Kanada, deals with ontology, i.e. the branch of metaphysics dealing with the nature of being. Vaiśeṣika derives its name from viśeṣ, which has different meanings such as 'characteristic', 'distinguishing', etc. Vaiśeṣika darśana deals with the knowledge of padārtha (objects). Padārtha is anything that can be denoted by a word, meaning it is namable. Vaiśeṣiks said that anything that has a name is real. Vaiśeṣika Darśana propounds two important aspects - one, of describing fundamental substances (padārtha), and two, the atomic model of the universe.

According to Kanada, the real is that which is knowable and nameable. By a subtle process of analysis and synthesis, Kanada divides all namables into six classes., viz., substance (dravya), attribute (guṇa), action (karma), genus (sāmānya), species (viśeṣa) and combination (samavāyānām). There is a seventh entity named abhāv. Abhāv means absence. Vaiśeṣika and Vedānta considers abhāv to be a positive knowledge of negation, and cannot be equated with knowledge through our senses. Vedānta later takes it up as an important method of knowledge in spiritual studies.

Padārtha

Āyurved's classification and understanding of drugs through their inherent rasa (taste), and study of the effect of drugs based on the guṇa (quality) is based on the knowledge of padārtha. Caraka Saṃhita mentions fifty-seven combinations and sixty-three types of variations of rasa according to dravya, (substance), place and time. Dravya, guṇa and karma are enumerated into further categories as below:

a. Dravya - Substance is further resolved into nine kinds: earth (pṛthvi), water (āpās), fire (tejas), air (vāyu), space (ākāśa), time (kāla), direction (dik), soul (atma) and mind (manas). Of these, the first four, earth, water, fire and air are wholes made up of parts which are non-eternal; whereas the last four, i.e. space, time, soul and mind are wholes without parts and therefore eternal.

b. Guṇa - Attributes are further divided into form (rūpa), taste (rasa), smell (gandha), touch (sparśa), numbers (sāṃkhya), measures (parimānāni), separateness (pṛthaktvatas), conjunction and disjunction (samyōg-vibhagau), priority and posteriority (paratvāparatve), understandings (buddhayah), pleasure and pain (sukha-dukhe), desire and aversion (ichcha-dveṣam), and volitions (prayatnah).

c. Karma - Action is further divided into throwing upwards (utkṣepaṇam), throwing downwards (avakṣepaṇam), contraction (ākuñcanam), expansion (prasāranam) and motion/going (gamanam).

The above three, i.e. substance, attributes and action are existent and non-eternal and have substance as their combinative cause, are effect as well as cause, and are both genus and species.

Vaiśeṣika also talks of how the soul can attain mokṣa from worldly existence through knowledge of the self. Kanada's fundamental teaching therefore is "tatva-jñānata-nihsreyasam" meaning, the supreme good results from the truth in the knowledge about the Soul. Kanada's philosophy shows how the Soul is to be known by distinguishing it from the material body.

Atomic theory of Vaiśeṣika

Vaiśeṣika provides the details of the atomic theory of creation by proposing the mahābhūtas of earth, water, fire and air as the basic building blocks of the universe (ether is not considered here), which have their individual characteristic and are distinguished from one another. These are the elemental substances or bhūta-dravya, which singly or by combination among themselves become the material causes of all products in the universe. This, say the Vaiśeṣika, account for the variety in nature. He refers to these as 'ultimate atoms' which are indivisible. The attributes of each mahābhūta is as follows

a. Earth has the attributes of form/colour (rūpa), taste (rasa), smell (gandha) and touch (sparśa)
b. Water possesses colour (rūpa), taste (rasa) and touch (sparśa), and are fluid and viscid
c. Fire possesses touch (sparśa) and colour (rūpa)
d. Air possess touch (sparśa)
e. None of the above characteristics belong to ether

Vaiśeṣika philosophy refuted the Sāṃkhya philosophy which said that prakṛti (matter) is the prime cause and established that ultimate atoms are the prime cause, and that they are eternal (indestructible).

Two primary atoms produce the binary (dvyaṇuka), which is still minute (aṇu) for it is without magnitude in the technical sense; three binaries produce the tryaṇuka (triad), in which form it can be perceived.

Law of Causation

The eternal (nityam), or that which cannot be annihilated is defined by Vaiśeṣika as sat (that which is existent) and akāranavat (not having a precedent cause). The existence of colour, etc. in the effect follows from its existence in the cause, i.e. the primary cause (ultimate atoms). He refutes the view that all is non-eternal and that there is nothing which is eternal. It is an error to assume that because things (ex. atoms) exist as effects (ex. compound bodies), therefore they cannot exist in the causal (or atomic) state.

When does an atom become perceptible?

An object becomes perceptible externally if it possesses magnitude by means of its possession of that which is composed of more than one substance and by means of its colour. The ultimate atoms have no magnitude and hence cannot be perceived.

In answer to what can be perceived, he says that numbers, magnitudes, separateness, conjunction and disjunction, priority and posteriority, and action become objects of visual perception, through their combination with substances possessing colour. If substances do not possess colour, they are not objects of visual perception. A mutual conjunction of the ultimate atoms as conditional causes of one another, is the possible way in which a body becomes perceptible.

The initial upward flaming of fire, the initial sideward blowing of air, the initial action of atoms and of mind, are caused by adṛṣṭam (consequences of actions in previous births). At the beginning of creation, action or motion arises in the ultimate atoms in consequence only of the conjunction of the soul carrying with it the invisible (adṛṣṭam) consequences of its previous acts, and the ultimate atoms, having by that action come together, originate in the order of binary atomic aggregate, etc.

Gravity

Gravity is defined as the non-inherent cause of the first movement of a falling body. The movement created by gravity produces velocity, which produces a second movement, of which the non-inherent cause is the first. Gravity is possessed of earth and water, and is super-sensible, and thus must be inferred.

Liberation

Pleasure and pain result from contact of the soul, sense, mind and object. For liberation, both pleasure and pain are to be freed from one's realm of experience. Mokṣa (spiritual liberation) consists in the non-existence of conjunction with the body, when at the same time, no potential body existing, and consequently, re-birth cannot take place.

Source:

1. Lecture on Vaiśeṣika Philosophy by Swami Samarpananda, Indian Spiritual Heritage
2. Sinha, Nandalal. The Sacred Book of the Hindus, The Vaisesika Sutra of Kanada, Vol VI, 1923
3. Keith, A.B. Indian Logic and Atomism: An exposition of the Nyaya and Vaisheshika systems, 1921
4. Seal, Brajendranath. The Positive Sciences of the Ancient Hindus, 1915

2

DHĀTU

Description of formation of the dhātu

Āyurved recognizes seven tissue layers called dhātu. The description of each dhātu and how it is formed and the problems that can occur at the level of each dhātu is given below:

1. **Rasa dhātu** or the lymph chyle exercises a soothing effect upon the entire organism and tends to contribute to the increased formation of blood. The loss of lymph chyle is marked by pain about the region of the heart, Angina Pectoris, with palpitation of the heart, a sensation of emptiness or gone-feeling in the viscus, and thirst. Increased germination of lymph chyle (rasa) in the body is manifest by such characteristics as, nausea, water-brash, and an increased flow of salivary secretion.
2. **Rakta dhātu** or blood, in its turn, increases the healthful glow of the complexion, leads to the increased formation of flesh and muscles and maintains vitality in the organism. The loss of blood is attended with such symptoms as roughness of the skin, and a craving for sour/acid food or drink. The patient longs to be in a cool place and asks for cool things, and the veins become

loose and flabby. Whereas, a plethora of blood in the system gives a reddish glow to the complexion and the white of the eyes, and imparts fullness to the veins.

3. **Mamsa dhātu** or the flesh contributes towards the stoutness or rotundity of the limbs and occasions the formation of fatty matter in the system. The loss of flesh is marked by emaciation of the buttocks, cheeks, lips, thighs, breasts, armpits, neck, and the calves of the legs. The arteries seem loose and flabby, and the body seems to be dry and inert, accompanied by an aching or gnawing pain in its members. An increase of flesh is marked by the rotundity and fullness of the buttocks and the lips, as well as of the penis, arms, and the thighs, and an increased heaviness of the whole body.

4. **Medha dhātu** or the fat gives rise to the glossiness (formation of oily or albuminous matter) of the body and primarily contributes towards the firmness and growth of the bones. The loss of fat is followed by such symptoms as the enlargement of the spleen, a sense of emptiness in the joints, and a peculiar dryness of the skin and a craving for cold and emollient meat. An excess of fat in the body imparts an oily gloss to the skin. The sides of the abdomen are increased in bulk, and the body emits a fetid smell, and the person is assailed with cough and dyspnoea.

5. **Asthi dhātu** or the bones, in their turn, support the body, and contribute to the formation of marrow. The degeneration of the bones is marked by an aching pain in the bones and bone-joints, a wasting of teeth and gums, and a general dryness of the body. An excessive

formation of bone (abnormal ossification) is attended with such symptoms as the cutting of additional teeth and the abnormal development of any of the bone-structures.

6. **Majja dhātu** or the marrow contributes towards the formation and increase of semen, and fills in the internal cavities of the bones, and forms the chief source of strength, amorous feelings and hilarity. The loss or waste of marrow is characterized by the formation of a lesser quantity of semen, aching pain in the bones and breaking pain in the bone-joints which would have become marrowless. An excessive formation of marrow gives rise to a heaviness of the eyes and to the members of the body.

7. **Śukra dhātu** or the semen gives rise to valour and courageousness, makes a man amorously disposed towards the female sex, increases his strength and amativeness, is the sole impregnating principle in the male organism, and is possessed of the virtue of being quickly emitted. The loss or waste of semen is marked by pain in the penis and the testes, and by incapacity for sexual intercourse. In such cases the emission of semen but rarely happens, and is then perceptibly deficient in its quantity, the emitted matter consisting of a small quantity of semen marked with shreds of blood. An excess of semen in the body is marked by an excessive flow of that fluid and gives rise to the formation of gravels (concretions) in the bladder which are known as śukraśmari.

In the case of loss or waste of the catamenial flow, the menses do not appear at the appointed time or are scanty. The vagina seems stuffed and painful. The medical treatment in such cases consists in the adoption of alterative or cleansing measures, and in the administration of drugs of a heat-making (āgneya) potency or virtue. An excess in the quantity of catamenial blood gives rise to an aching of the limbs and an excessive flow.

The highest stage to which food attains is the semen/ ovum, which takes about one month. Śukra is the seventh and final dhātu as a sāra (essence) of all dhātu and produced in a progressive evolutive metamorphosis.

8. **Oja dhatu** - The quintessence of all the fundamental principles of the body, starting with lymph chyle and ending with semen/ovum, is called the Ojas, which is identical with what is termed "vital power." The whole body with its limbs and members is permeated with Ojas, and a loss or diminution in its natural quantity leads to the gradual emaciation (and ultimate dissolution) of the organism. A blow, a persistent wasting disease, anger, grief, cares and anxieties, fatigue and hunger, are the causes to which should be ascribed the wasting or disappearance of this strength-giving principle (albumen) of the body.

Source:

Kaviraj Kunja Lal Bhishagratna, An English Translation of Suśruta Saṃhita. Vol I, Suthrasthanam, Chapter Chapter XIV: Shonita-Varnaniya-Madhyayam

3

PAÑCAMAHĀBHŪTA

Description of pañca mahābhūtas as per Āyurved

The five fundamental principles which are earth (pṛthvi), water (āpās), fire (agni), air (vāyu) and sky (ākāśa) enter into the composition of all substances in the world, and the predominance of any of them in a particular substance determines its character.

1. **Earth principle** - A substance, which is thick, pithy, compact, dull, immobile, rough, heavy (hard to digest), strong smelling and largely has a sweet taste marked by a shade of astringent, is called a substance of dominant earth (pārthivam) matter. Such a substance increases the firmness, strength, hardness and rotundity of the human body, and is possessed of gravity (the virtue of moving the bowels).

2. **Water principle** - A substance, which is cold, moist, glossy, devoid of keenness, takes time to be digested, is mobile, compact, soft, slimy, sappy, and is largely endued with an acid, saline or sweet taste marked by a shade of astringent, is called a substance of dominant water (āpyam) principle. Such a thing soothes and imparts a

glossy character to the body, keeps it moist, favours the adhesion of its parts, and increases its liquid contents.

3. **Fire principle** - A substance, which is heat-making, pungent and keen, subtle in its essence, permeates the minutest capillaries, and is dry, rough, light, and non-slimy in its character and has strong properties and a taste which is largely pungent marked by a shade of saline, is called a substance of the dominant principle of fire (taijasam). Such a thing naturally evinces an up-coursing tendency in the body, produces a burning sensation in its inside, helps the process of digestion and spontaneous bursting (of abscesses), increases the temperature of the body, strengthens the eyesight, improves the complexion and imparts a healthful glow to it.

4. **Air principle** - A substance, which is subtle in its essence, and is dry, rough, light, cold and non- slimy, increases tactual sensation and is endued with a largely astringent taste marked by a shade of bitter, is called a substance of the dominant principle of air (vāyaviyam). Such a thing removes the slimy character of the internal organism, produces lightness, dryness and emaciation of the body, and increases the speculative or contemplative faculty of mind.

5. **Ether principle** - A substance, which is smooth, unctuous, and is subtle in its nature, soft or pliant in its consistency, expansive in the internal organism, porous, sound-making and non-slimy in its character without

any definite taste, is called a substance of the dominant principle of ether (ākashiyam). Such a substance produces softness, lightness and porosity of the body.

Source:

Kaviraj Kunja Lal Bhishagratna, An English Translation of Suśruta Saṃhita. Vol I, Suthrasthana. Chapter XLI, Dravya-Vishesha-Vijnaniya-Madhyamam.

4

SUB TYPES OF DOṢA

Description of five sub-types of vāta doṣa

The five types of vāta doṣa according to their functions and locations are Prāṇa, Udāna, Vyāna, Samāna and Apāna. Their descriptions are given below:

1. **Prāṇa Vayu** —The vāyu that courses in (governs) the cavity of the mouth is called the prāṇa. Its function being to force down the food into the cavity of the stomach, and to assist the different vitalizing principles of the body such as the internal heat or fire etc. in discharging their functions in life, and to contribute to the general sustenance of the body. A deranged condition of prāṇa vāyu is usually followed by hiccough, dyspnea and other similar distempers. Prāṇa vāyu is identical with the energy of the nerve centre in the medulla. (this is not to be confused with Prāṇa which is the vital life force, and the meanings should be derived based on the context of using the word)

2. **Udāna Vayu** - The vāyu which courses upward, is called the Udāna. It produces speech, song, etc. In its deranged state it brings on diseases which are specifically confined to regions lying above the clavicles.

3. **Samāna vāyu** - The samāna vāyu governs the stomach (āmāśaya) and the region of intestines (pakvaśaya). Its functions consist in digesting the chyme brought down into the intestines in unison with the digestive fire (agni), and especially in disintegrating its essence from its refuse or excreted matter. A deranged or aggravated condition of the Samāna vāyu causes dysentery, gulma, and impaired digestion, etc. The samāna is same as the energy of the epigastric plexus.

4. **Vyāna vāyu** - The vāyu known as the Vyāna courses (acts) through the whole organism, and its functions consist in sending the lymph chyle etc. all through the body and in helping the out-flow of blood and perspiration. Five kinds of muscular movements are ascribed to the action of the Vyāna vāyu, a deranged condition of which is generally attended with diseases which are not confined to any particular region, member, or organ of the body, but are found to affect the whole organism (such as, fever, etc). The five actions are expansion, flexion, lowering down and lifting up or lateral thrusting of any part of the body. Vyāna is same as the energy of the motor-sensory nerves.

5. **Apāna vāyu** —The vāyu known as the Apāna acts in the lower region of the intestines (pakvādhāna). Its functions consist in bearing down the foetus and the faeces and in evacuating the urine, semen and menstrual blood. An enraged condition of this vāyu tends to bring on serious diseases, which are peculiar to the urinary bladder and the distal portion of the large intestine (guda). An aggravated condition of both the vyāna and apāna vāyu

may produce prameha (diabetes) and disorders of the seminal fluid. The apāna is identical with the force of the hypogastric plexus. (Heat and a burning sensation in the affected part and a profuse menorrhagia mark a case when the apāna vāyu becomes surcharged with the pitta).

Description of five sub-types of pitta doṣa

The five types of pitta doṣa according to their functions and locations are Pācaka, Rañjaka, Sādhaka, Ālocaka and Bhrājaka. Their descriptions are given below:

1. **Pācakāgni** – The heat of digestion, which is situated in the region between the stomach and the intestines; and being a liquid fire or fluid heat incarcerated in the secretions of the liver (bile), it is primarily concerned in digesting the four kinds of food (as they meet it in the abdomen). It is this pitta, which makes metabolism in other parts of the body possible, helping the organism in acquiring fresh energy.
2. **Rañjaka** - The second kind of pitta is called rañjaka or pigment pitta from the circumstance of its imparting the characteristic colour to the lymph chyle as it is transformed into blood by coursing through the liver and spleen, where it is located.
3. **Sādhaka** - The third kind of pitta is called **sādhaka** and is situated in the heart. It indirectly assists in the performance of cognitive functions in man by keeping up the rhythmic cardiac contractions. Its actions also bring about a fruition or realization of one's desires.

4. **Ālocaka** - The fourth, which is the **ālocaka** or the pittam of sight; indicates the metabolic process in the substance of the retina (dṛṣṭi) which gives rise to visual sensation.
5. **Bhrājakāgni** - The fifth is the **bhrājakāgni** or the pitta in the skin which produces perspiration or helps exudations from the skin by evaporation. In short it is the pitta which keeps active, under certain circumstances, the secretions from the sweat and sebaceous glands of the human skin.

Description of five sub-types of kapha doṣa

The five types of kapha doṣa according to their functions and locations are Kledaka, Avalamvaka, Vodhakam, Tarpakam and Śleṣmakam. Their descriptions are given below:

1. **Kledaka** - The kapha, even though principally located in the stomach, permeates its four other distant localities with its peculiar watery or humid essence in virtue of its inherent attributes.
2. **Avalamvaka** - The kapha, located in the region of the chest, protects the joints of the arms, the neck and the sternum, and enables the heart to perform its natural functions with the help of the lymph-chyle derived from the assimilated food and its own intrinsic potency.
3. **Vodhakam** —The kapha, situated in the throat and at the root of the palate, lends its aid to the perception of tastes by maintaining the moist or humid character of the tongue.

4. **Tarpakam** —The kapha, situated in the head, cools and bathes the different sense organs with its own humid essence, in virtue of its natural humid attributes.

5. **Śleṣmakam** - The kapha, situated in the joints, keeps them firmly united, protects their articulation and opposes their separation and disunion.

Source: Kaviraj Kunja Lal Bhishagratna, An English Translation of Suśruta Saṃhita. Vol I, Suthrasthana, Chapter XXI - Vrana-prashna-madhyayam

5

ṢAT RASA – THE SIX TASTES

The six types of Rasa (tastes), and their properties are given below:

1. **Madhura** (sweet) – A taste, which is pleasant, proves comfortable to, and contributes to the life-preservation of a man, keeps his mouth moist, and increases the quantity of bodily kapham, is called madhura. The main characteristics of madhura rasa are given below:
   - Pañcamahābhūta – pṛthvi (earth) and āpās (water)
   - Subdues doṣa – vāyu, pitta
   - Hot/Cold – Cooling property
   - Character – Heavy and emollient
   - Examples – Ghee, thickened milk, lard, śālī rice (red rice), ṣāṣṭika rice, yava (barley), godhuma (wheat), māṣa pulse (black gram), sugarcane, kuṣmāṇḍa (ash gourd), trāpusa (cucumber), gourds, etc.

2. **Amla** (acid/sour) - A taste, which produces tooth-edge and increased salivation, and increases the relish for food, is called amla. The main characteristics of amla rasa are given below:

- Pañcamahābhūta – pṛthvi (earth) and agni (fire)
- Subdues doṣa – vāyu
- Hot/Cold – Heating property
- Character – Heavy and emollient
- Examples – gooseberry, curd, whey, pomegranate, citron, wood apple, lime, vinegar, jujube, dhānyāmla (sour gruel made from the fermentation of rice water), rice gruel

3. Lavaṇa (saline) - A taste, which imparts a greater relish to food, produces salivation and softness of a part, is called lavaṇa. The main characteristics of lavaṇa rasa are given below:
    - Pañcamahābhūta – āpās (water) and agni (fire)
    - Subdues doṣa - vāyu
    - Hot/Cold – Heating property
    - Character – Heavy and emollient
    - Examples – salt, black salt, yavakṣāra (nitrate of potash), etc.
4. **Kaṭuka** (pungent) - A taste, which produces a burning sensation on the tip of the tongue attended with a tingling of the part and headache, and is instantaneously followed by a running at the nose (fluent coryza) is called kaṭuka/kaṭu. The main characteristics of kaṭuka rasa are given below:
    - Pañcamahābhūta – vāyu (air) and agni (fire)
    - Subdues doṣa – kapha
    - Hot/Cold – Heating property
    - Character – Dry and Light

- ✦ Examples – Pepper, drumstick, radish, garlic, camphor, pine, etc.

5. **Tikta** (bitter) - A taste, which gives rise to a sort of sucking sensation in the throat, removes the slimy character of the cavity of the mouth, gives rise to the appearance of goose-flesh on the skin, and increases the relish for food, is called tikta. The main characteristics of tikta rasa are given below:

   - ✦ Pañcamahābhūta – vāyu (air) and ākāśa (ether)
   - ✦ Subdues doṣa - pitta, kapha
   - ✦ Hot/Cold – Cooling property
   - ✦ Character – Dry and Light
   - ✦ Examples – bamboo shoot, turmeric, neem, bitter-gourd, eggplant, ashoka tree, etc

6. **Kaṣāya** (astringent) – A taste, which brings about the dryness of the mouth, numbs the palate, obstructs the throat, and gives rise to a drawing, pressing sensation in the region of the heart, is called kaṣāya. The main characteristics of Kaṣāya rasa are given below:

   - ✦ Pañcamahābhūta – pṛthvi (earth) and vāyu (air)
   - ✦ Subdues doṣa – pitta, kapha
   - ✦ Hot/Cold – Cooling property
   - ✦ Character – Dry and Light
   - ✦ Examples - triphalā, cherry, kataka (clearing nut), pear, amaranth, chilli, methi (fenugreek), etc.

Specific Virtues of Tastes

1. **Madhura (Sweet)**

a) Increasing the quantity of lymph-chyle, blood, flesh, fat, bone marrow, albumen (ojas), semen/ovum, and milk in a parturient woman.

b) Contributes to the growth of bones, strengthens the eyesight, favours the growth of hair, improves the complexion of the body, brings about the adhesion of fractured bones (sandhānam), and purifies the blood and the lymph chyle.

c) Wholesome for infants, old and weak men and ulcer-patients

d) Exhilarates the mind as well as the five sense-organs, relieves thirst, swooning and a burning sensation of the body, and originates kapha.

e) Favours germination of intestinal parasites

f) If had in excess, sweet taste brings on cough, dyspnoea, flatulence (alasaka), vomiting, sweet taste in the mouth, hoarseness of the voice (aphonia), worms in the intestines, tumours, elephantisis, vasti-lepa (mucous deposit in the bladder), gudopolepa (mucous or slimy deposit in the anus), and abhisandya (ophthalmia), etc.

2. Amla (Acid/Sour)

a. An acid taste should be regarded as a digestant of assimilated food, and is endued with resolving, appetizing and carminative properties.

b. It sets in the natural emission of flatus and urine, restores the natural movements of the bowels, lessens the tendency to spasms, and gives rise to an acid (digestive) reaction in the stomach, and to a sensation of external shivering.

c. It originates a slimy or mucous secretion and is extremely pleasant or relishing.

d. An acid taste, though possessed of the aforesaid virtues, brings on tooth-edge, with sudden closing of the eyes, appearance of goose flesh on the skin, absorption of kapha and looseness of the body in the event of its being largely partaken of to the exclusion of all other tastes.

e. It gives rise to a burning sensation in the throat, chest and the region of the heart.

3. Lavaṇa (Saline)

a. A saline taste is possessed of corrective (purgative and emetic) virtues, favours the processes of suppuration and spontaneous bursting of swellings, brings about the looseness or resolution of any affected part (ulcer), is heat-engendering in its property and proves incompatible with all other tastes.

b. It cleanses the internal passages or channels of the organism and produces softness of the limbs and members of the body.

c. A saline taste, though possessed of the aforesaid properties, may bring on scabies

d. Urticaria, oedematous swellings, loss or discoloration of the natural complexion of the body, loss of virile potency, distressing symptoms affecting the sense-organs, inflammation of the mouth and the eyes, haemoptysis, vāta-rakta (a kind of leprosy) and acid eructation etc., in the event of its being largely partaken of to the exclusion of all other tastes.

4. Kaṭuka (Pungent)

a. A pungent taste is endued with appetising, resolving (pācana) and purifying properties in respect of ulcers etc., and destroys obesity, languor, deranged kapha and intestinal parasites.

b. It is antitoxic in its character, proves curative in cases of kuṣṭa (skin diseases) and itches, and removes the stiffness of the ligaments.

c. It acts as a sedative and reduces the quantity of semen, milk and fat

d. A pungent taste, though possessed of the aforesaid virtues, may bring on vertigo, loss of consciousness, dryness of the throat, palate and lips, burning sensation and a high temperature of the body, loss of strength, tremor, a sort of aching or breaking pain, and a neuralgic pain (vāta-śūla) in the back, sides and the extremities, etc. in the event of its being largely partaken of in exclusion of all other tastes.

5. Tikta (Bitter)

a. A bitter taste serves to restore the natural relish of a person for food and brings on a sense of general languor.

b. It is a good appetiser, and acts as a good purifying agent (in respect of ulcers, etc.), and proves curative in itches and urticaria.

c. It removes thirst, swoon and fever, purifies mother's milk, and is possessed of the virtue of drying up urine, ordure, mucous, fat and pus, etc.

d. A bitter taste, though possessed of the aforesaid properties, may bring on numbness of the limbs, wry-neck, convulsions, facial paralysis, violent headache, giddiness, and an aching, cutting and breaking pain, as well as a bad taste in the mouth in the event of its being largely partaken of in exclusion of all other tastes.

6. Kaṣāya (Astringent)

a. An astringent taste is possessed of astringent, healing, styptic (stambana), purifying, liquefacient, drying and contracting virtues.

b. It lessens secretions from mucous membranes.

c. An astringent taste, though possessed of the above said properties, may bring on the peculiar type of heart disease known as (hṛdroga) parchedness of the mouth, distention of the abdomen, loss of speech, wry-neck (mānya stamha), throbbing or quivering and tingling sensations in the body with contraction of the limbs and convulsions, etc.

Source:

Kaviraj Kunja Lal Bhishagratna, An English Translation of Suśruta Saṃhita. Vol I, Suthrasthana, Chapter XLII – Rasa-Vishesha-Vijnaniya-madhyayam

6

Ṣat Cakra – The Six Cakras

The six cakras, their properties with respect to the Annamaya Kosha (physical body) and corresponding regions of influence are given below:

1. Mūlādhāra cakra

Mūlā means root, and ādhāra means foundation. Mūlādhāra refers to the root of our being. This is the first or lower-most cakra, situated at the base of the spinal column.

Location: It is situated below the genitals and above the perineum.

Plexus: Mūlādhāra cakra corresponds to the coccygeal plexus and serves the region called the coccyx (also called tailbone, situated at the base of the spine).

Gland: Reproductive glands or Gonads

Doṣa: apāna vāyu

Element: Pṛthvī (earth)

Influence: Mūlādhāra corresponds to the functioning of basic instincts and survival processes. If the mūlādhāra cakra is not active or insufficiently energized, it will have an impact on basic life processes. Hence, emotions of fear, insecurity, distrust and a struggle to survive on a day-to-day basis are associated with an insufficiently energized mūlādhāra cakra. When people operate primarily from mūlādhāra cakra, their priorities in life will revolve around food, shelter and sexual activity. When mūlādhāra cakra is fully energized, the struggle to survive will diminish and people can move on to higher pursuits. It is said that in the Kali Yuga, most people operate from the mūlādhāra cakra and hence strengthening this cakra is essential for propelling people to go beyond basic survival.

Temples: Several temples in villages dedicated to the grāma devata (village deity) are consecrated to energize the mūlādhāra cakra, and provide a sense of protection and security to the people. The deity in these temples are often in the fierce form (ugra rūpa) or in a warrior pose wielding weapons. Such deities face the outside of the village/town away from where people live, offering protection to the people from enemies outside the village/town. These temples offer a sense of stability, wellbeing and harmony, by energizing or balancing the mūlādhāra cakra.

2. Svadhiṣṭhāna cakra

Sva means Self, and adhiṣṭhāna means seat. Svadhiṣṭhāna refers to the seat of the Supreme Self. It is where Śakti, the primordial feminine force, resides. This is the second cakra from the base of the spine.

Location: Root of the genitals

Plexus: Svadhiṣṭhāna cakra correspond to the sacral plexus that arise from the lower back just above the sacrum. The sacral plexus provides motor and sensory nerves for the pelvis, thigh, knee, calf and foot.

Gland: Ovaries in females and testes in males

Doṣa: apāna vāyu

Element: varuṇa/āpās (water)

Influence: Functions of the Svadhiṣṭhāna cakra are closely associated with functions of the mūlādhāra cakra. While mūlādhāra is largely associated with the basic survival, svadhiṣṭhāna is mainly associated with procreative abilities. When it is not sufficiently energized, it impacts the functioning of ovaries in women, thereby causing menstrual and reproductive health disorders. The mūlādhāra and svadhiṣṭhāna cakras are essential for proper functioning of the downward moving apāna vāyu which directs the flow of menstrual blood and aids the process of birthing. Any change in direction of apāna vāyu or blockages in its movement could result in menstrual and reproductive disorders for women.

Temples: Devī temples associated with fertility, are examples of temples that work to energize the Svadhiṣṭhāna cakra and rectify any alterations in the apāna vāyu, thereby resolving problems of infertility and other reproductive health issues. Such temples are often associated with ensuring good health, fertility and well-being.

3. Maṇipūra cakra

Maṇi refers to a precious gem, and pūra is the term used to denote a region or town. Therefore, maṇipūra refers to the land of the precious gem, indicating wealth and prosperity. This is the third cakra from the base of the spine.

Location: It is situated in the root/base of the navel

Plexus: Maṇipūra cakra corresponds to the region of the Solar plẹxus

Gland: Adrenal Glands and Pancreas

Doṣa: Samāna vāyu

Element: Agni (fire)

Influence: Maṇipūra cakra regulates the functions of digestion and assimilation of food. Energizing the maṇipūra cakra increases the digestive fire, pitta, which not only aids physical digestion of food, but also provides the fire power to pursue worldly goals. This cakra also regulates the samāna vāyu, which is responsible for digestion and assimilation of food. Those who are active in this cakra would often have an aggressive personality and an ambitious nature. This cakra provides the ambition and drive to do well in worldly affairs.

Temples: Temples which work to energize the maṇipūra cakra provide devotees in the pravṛtti mārg with the fire (agni) required to fulfill worldly desires and achieve materialistic goals. The element of agni is powerful in these temples. For those on the spiritual path, maṇipūra cakra is the start of the process of renunciation. The Umānanda temple in Guwahati (Assam) is an example where one can experience the spiritual aspects of this cakra.

4. Anāhata cakra

Anāhata refers to unstruck sound. That is, sound which is not produced by clanging of two objects.

Location: It is situated in the region of the heart.

Plexus: Anāhata cakra corresponds to the cardiac plexus.

Gland: Thymus gland

Doṣa: vyāna vāyu

Element: vāyu (air)

Influence: At the physical level, energizing the anāhata cakra takes the person towards a more compassionate and inclusive way of living, rather than being only materialistic. It also helps in dispelling fear. When this cakra is active, being kind and exuding compassion becomes effortless. Anāhata cakra influences the vyāna vāyu which is responsible for maintaining circulation and balancing the other vāyus in the body.

Temples: Temples that energize the anāhata cakra are powerful centres of overcoming fear and having desires fulfilled. Several Bhadrakāli and Durga temples trigger the anāhata cakra, removing the cause of fear and granting devotees their wishes.

5. Viśuddhi cakra

Viśuddhi means highly pure or a purifying filter.

Location: It is situated in the region of the neck, at the base of the throat.

Plexus: It corresponds to the cervical plexus which governs the regions of neck, head and shoulders. It also corresponds to the region of the pharynx and larynx, and therefore, the pharyngeal and laryngeal plexus.

Gland: Thyroid and Parathyroid gland

Doṣa: udāna vāyu

Element: ākāśa (space/ether)

Influence: At the physical level, activation of the viśuddhi cakra helps with problems pertaining to the thyroid gland and the throat region. Improved speech, articulation and creativity are associated with this cakra. Viśuddhi cakra also influences the role of the udāna vāyu which is responsible for exhalation and speech.

Temples: Temples that energize the viśuddhi cakra work as a gateway for the great liberation. Once this cakra is active, there is no going back, and the pathway for mukti is laid. Srikalahasthi temple in Andhra Pradesh is a popular Śakta viśuddhi kṣetram.

6. Ājñā cakra

Ājñā literally means command. One in whom the ājñā cakra is active, has command over his/her mind.

Location: It is situated in the region between the eyebrows, also called the third eye.

Plexus: This cakra corresponds to the Carotid plexus and the Cavernous plexus.

Gland: Pituitary gland and the hypothalamus

Doṣa: prāṇa vāyu

Element: ākāśa (space/ether)

Influence: At the physical level, the pituitary gland and hypothalamus are the command centres for the rest of the endocrine glands. Therefore, energizing this cakra is necessary for all hormones, including growth and reproductive hormones, to function appropriately. When this cakra is inactive, functions pertaining to these glands are affected. On a spiritual level, ājñā cakra activation helps devotees move closer to the spiritual union with the divine. Ājñā cakra also influences the prāṇa vāyu which is responsible for inhalation and pushing down of ingested food.

Temples: Temples that energize the ājñā cakra work to stimulate the pituitary and its functions on a physical level. Most of the popular temples such as Sabarimala and many Śiva temples are meant to activate the ājñā cakra and assist devotees in the spiritual path.

Source: Joseph, Sinu. 'Women and Sabarimala: Science behind Restrictions', Notionpress, 2019

INDEX

A

Ādāna kāla 209

Adhmāna 97

Advaita vedānta 37

Āgama 26, 30, 32, 239, 259

Āgama śāstra 26, 30, 259

Agni 50, 95, 114, 187, 207, 210–213, 272, 291, 332, 357, 361, 366, 375

Ājñā 272, 274, 277–278, 281, 302, 377–378

Ājñā cakra 277–278, 281, 302, 377–378

Ākāśa 50, 95, 210, 272, 332, 349, 357, 367, 376–377

Amāvāsyā 175, 177–180, 184–185, 268–269

Ambubachi 214, 285–292, 297, 310

Amla 95, 114, 210–211, 365, 368

Anāhata 272, 274–275, 278, 281, 375–376

Anāhata cakra 272, 375–376

Anavasthitatva 110

Antina unde 77

Aṇu 50, 350

Anulepana 119

Anumāna 48, 332, 338, 343

Anupacaya 188–189, 191–192, 194–195

Anupacaya sthāna 188, 192, 194–195

Anyamata-parīkṣā 343

Āpā 95, 212

Apāna 127, 156–157, 164, 205, 246–250, 268, 325–327, 335, 360

Apāna 127, 156–157, 164, 205, 246–250, 268, 325–327, 335, 360

Apāna vāyu 156, 164, 246–250, 268, 325–327

Āpās 50, 332, 349, 357, 365–366, 374

Āptavacana 48, 332, 338

Ārati 77, 81

Ārṣa 241

Ārtava 105–106

Āṣāḍha 291

Asthi 108, 114, 354

Atharva 55

Avayava 343, 345

Ayana 180

Āyurved 11, 17, 30, 32, 37–38, 45–51, 53–59, 64–65, 73, 75, 78, 92, 94–98, 105–109, 113–114, 117, 122, 124, 129, 131, 133, 136–137, 140, 145, 151, 153–156, 158, 160–161, 165–166, 174, 178, 205–209, 217, 256, 311, 318, 331, 333, 340, 342, 344, 346, 348, 353, 357

B

Bagalamukhī 289

Bala 96, 212–215, 217

Balya 96, 98

Bhagavathi 33, 134, 234, 264

Bhagvan 228, 313

Bhairavī 289

Bhakti 34

Bharatanatyam 150

Bhuja 239

Bhukti 246–247, 249, 259, 290, 308, 318

Bhūr 276, 280–281

Bhūr 276, 280–281

Bhūta-dravya 50, 350

Bhuva 280–281

Bhuvaneśvarī 289

Bindi 81

Brāhma-hatya 313

Brahman 226, 229–230, 289, 306, 309

Brāhmaṇa 32, 313–315

Brahma-pīṭha 304

Brahmi 307

Brihat jātaka 179, 187–188

Bṛṃhaṇa 96, 98

C

Caitanyam 227, 229, 232, 237–238, 241, 243, 247, 261, 265, 267, 270, 308

Cakras 12, 224, 234, 242–243, 246–249, 272, 274–275, 277–278, 280–281, 283, 295, 301–302, 308, 316, 325–327, 372, 374

Cakras. 12, 234, 242–243, 246–247, 249, 272, 274–275, 280–281, 301–302, 326, 374

Candra mās 177

Caraka 42, 49, 55–57, 64, 67, 105, 109, 132, 209, 213, 333, 348

Caraka saṃhita 49, 105, 132, 348

Caraka saṃhitā 42, 49, 57, 67, 109, 333
Chalam 346
Chandra-rāśi 188, 192
Chaupadi 34, 147
Chengannur bhagavathy 12, 262, 269, 285
Chinnamasta 289
Cikitsā 169

D

Dadiyamu 80
Daivika 241
Dakṣiṇāyana 180, 209, 291, 311
Dakṣiṇāyana 180, 209, 291, 311
Danta 275
Darbha 92
Darśana 12, 32, 48–49, 51, 224, 229, 231, 331, 340, 343, 348
Daśa mahā vidyās 289, 306
Devata 228–229, 373
Devī 31, 33, 134, 179, 214, 226, 228, 230–231, 234, 237–238, 243, 246–247, 261, 263–268, 285–289, 299, 301, 303–307, 374
Dhaniṣṭha 194
Dhāraṇā 49, 341
Dhātu 12, 96, 107–108, 114, 123, 132, 136, 300, 318, 342, 353–356
Dhātu 12, 96, 107–108, 114, 123, 132, 136, 300, 318, 342, 353–356
Dhūmavati 289
Dhvaja-stambha 241
Dhyān 49, 341
Dhyān 49, 341
Dhyāna 224
Doṣa 12, 56, 95–97, 107, 109–112, 114–116, 119, 121–123, 125, 132–133, 136, 151–153, 156, 158, 160, 162, 164–165, 171, 204–207, 209–214, 244–245, 291, 360, 362–363, 365–367, 372, 374–377
Dravatva 114
Dṛṣṭāntata 345
Durga 261, 307, 376
Dvāpara yuga 223
Dvyaṇuka 346, 350

G

Gala 239
Gati 109
Gauṇa 75–76
Gaurava 119
Gayatri mantra 250, 275–278, 280–281
Gharṣaṇa 96
Gochara 190, 193
Golla 141–143, 145–147, 149

Graha 177, 189
Grāma devathā 247
Grīṣma 209, 211, 213, 215, 217, 291
Guhyamahābhairavi 231
Guṇa 49, 348–349
Guñjā 105
Guruji 5, 236–237

H

Haviṣya-anna 78
Hemanta 209–210, 212–215, 217
Hetvabhāsa 345
Hora 189–190, 193–195, 201
Hosige 77

I

Icchā 230
Indrā 32
Iṣṭa devata 228–229

J

Jalpah 345
Janah 280–281
Jātih 346
Jñāna 259, 340
Jyeṣṭhā 291
Jyotiṣa śāstra 32, 175–176, 187–190, 201

K

Kajal 118, 132
Kalari cikitsā 169
Kalaripayattu 150–151, 165–169
Kāli 179, 231, 261, 289, 306–307
Kali yuga 223, 225–226, 373
Kāli. 306
Kālika purāna 304–306
Kāma 296, 314–315
Kāmākhya 12, 31, 34, 134, 214, 236, 247, 266, 285–286, 288–292, 295–296, 298–310
Kapha 50, 56, 59, 95, 97–98, 107, 109, 118–122, 152, 206, 210–211, 214, 363–364, 366–370
Kapha 50, 56, 59, 95, 97–98, 107, 109, 118–122, 152, 206, 210–211, 214, 363–364, 366–370
Kapham 109, 365
Kāraka 177
Karṇa 239
Kaṭī 239
Kaṭuka 95, 366, 370
Katyayini 307
Khichidi 82, 88–89, 98
Kośa 21, 73–74
Krishna kuteer 146
Kriyā 259
Kumbha 192, 194, 196–198, 200, 203

Kuṇḍali 231

Kundalini 273, 294

Kuṅkuma 81, 140, 300

Kushti 166, 169

L

Laghu 109, 210

Lagna 188–189, 191

Lakṣmī 228, 303, 307

Lavana 95

M

Madhura 95–97, 119, 210–212, 365, 368

Madhura 95–97, 119, 210–212, 365, 368

Mahābhūtas 50, 209, 332, 346, 350, 357

Mahah 280–281

Mahāpīṭha 304

Majjā 108

Māṃsa 96, 108, 299

Māṃsa dhātu 96

Maṅgal snān 81–82

Maṇipūra 247–248, 272, 275, 278, 280–281, 294–295, 299, 311, 374–375

Maṇipūra 247–248, 272, 275, 278, 280–281, 294–295, 299, 311, 374–375

Manobhava-guhā 305

Manomaya kośa 73–74

Mantra japa 248

Mantra vidyā 272

Mantras 12, 31, 246, 250, 272, 275–278, 305, 309

Mānuṣa 241

Marma cikitsā 169

Mārtsnya 119

Māyā 231, 286, 311

Meda dhātu 96

Medas 108

Melsanthi 264

Melśānti 229, 263–264, 269, 271

Meṣa 188, 190, 192–193, 196–198, 200, 203

Mīmāmsā darśana 231

Mīna 188, 190, 192, 196–198, 200, 203

Mokṣa dham 249, 254

Mukha 239

Mukti 246–247, 249, 259, 290, 298–299, 304, 306, 309–310, 316–319, 336, 377

Mūlādhāra 234, 243, 247–248, 272–275, 278, 280–281, 372–374

Mūlādhāra 234, 243, 247–248, 272–275, 278, 280–281, 372–374

Mūlāprakrti 231

Mūrddhā 275

Mūrti 226, 236–239, 241, 286

N

Nāḍīparīkṣā 64
Nāḍīs 242–243, 274
Nakhābheda 113
Nakṣatra mās 177
Nakṣatras 176, 189, 198–199
Nālanda 60
Narasimhi 307
Nāsikā 239
Navayōni 304
Nigrahasthānam 346
Nirguṇa 226
Nirṇaya 345
Nisumbha 307
Nyāya 48–49, 64, 331, 343–344, 346–347

O

Om prati-tiṣṭha parameśvara 238
Oṣṭha 275

P

Pāda 239, 259
Padārtha 49, 348
Padma-purāṇa 241
Paicchilya 119
Pañca mahābhūta 59
Pañcamahābhūta 12, 95, 272, 357, 365–367
Pandit 223, 229
Paramāṇu 50
Pārvati 231, 304
Paschimottāsana 325
Paschimottāsana 325
Pasupu theertham 81
Paurānas 241
Perantam 81–82
Pīṭha 236, 304
Pitta 45, 50, 56, 59, 78, 95–98, 107, 109, 114–119, 121–122, 124–126, 128–129, 132–133, 152, 158, 166, 168, 187, 207–208, 211–214, 291, 362–363, 365, 367, 375
Pitta prakopa 115–117, 152
Pragjyotiṣapura 291
Prakopa 111–113, 115–117, 120–122, 152, 165
Pramāṇa 46, 49, 333, 338, 343–344
Pramāṇas 48–49, 332–333
Prameya 344
Prāṇa 25, 58–59, 73, 94, 124–127, 225–227, 238, 241, 243–245, 247–248, 259, 310, 335, 360, 377–378
Prāṇa 25, 58–59, 73, 94, 124–127, 225–227, 238, 241, 243–245, 247–248, 259, 310, 335, 360, 377–378
Prāṇa pratiṣṭha 25
Prāṇa vidyā 94

Prāṇamaya kośa 73–74
Prāṇāyāma 33, 138, 186
Prāṇāyāma 45
Prasāra 230
Pratyāhāra 341
Pratyakṣa 46, 48, 332, 338, 343
Pratyakṣa pramāṇa 46
Prayojana 344
Pṛthvi 50, 95, 212, 272, 332, 349, 357, 365–367
Pūjā 80, 82, 224, 229, 248, 252–253, 255–256, 263, 299
Pūjāri 229, 271
Purāṇa 17, 223, 241, 311–312, 321
Pūrṇimā 175, 178–180, 184–185, 269
Puruṣa 59, 224, 229, 320, 331–333, 335–337

R

Rajah-srāva-kāla 205
Rajasic 319
Rajaswala 108–109, 129–130, 133, 319
Rajaswala paricaryā 108–109, 133
Rakta 56, 108, 305, 353, 369
Rasa 12, 49–50, 95–97, 107–108, 117, 123, 209–212, 331, 348–350, 353, 365–367, 371
Rāśi 188, 190–194, 199
Raudri 307
Ṛgveda saṃhitā 276
Ṛṣis 49, 223
Ṛtu cakra 204, 213
Ṛtu kāla saṃskāra 76
Ṛtu vyatīta kāla 207
Rudrapīṭha 304
Rūkṣatā 109

S

Sabarimala 17, 34, 249–250, 254, 257–258, 261, 263–264, 269–271, 290, 295, 309, 311, 321, 378
Ṣaḍ-darśana 32, 48
Sadh 224
Sādhana 78, 206, 223–224, 234, 251, 282, 289, 309–310, 317–320
Sahasrāra 234, 243, 281
Sahasrāra cakra 243
Śakti 72, 135, 226, 229–232, 247, 274, 288, 299, 304, 306, 373
Samādhi 223
Samādhi 49, 341
Samādhi 49, 341
Samāna 245–246, 325, 335, 360–361, 375
Saṃhita 49, 65, 97, 105–106, 132, 209, 241, 321, 348, 356, 359, 364, 371

Saṃhita 49, 65, 97, 105–106, 132, 209, 241, 321, 348, 356, 359, 364, 371
Sāṃkhya darśana 48–49, 229, 331
Saṃśaya 339, 344
Saṃskṛtam 15, 56, 209, 222, 238, 272, 274–275, 324, 326, 331, 337
Samurta 78
Saṃyama 49, 341–342
Saṅkalpa 227
Śānti pūjā 80
Śaradā 209, 212–213, 217
Śāstra 17, 24–26, 30, 32, 175–176, 187–190, 201, 223–227, 232, 239, 259, 272, 343
Ṣat cakra 12, 372
Ṣat rasa 12, 95, 117, 365
Sattva 319, 321, 333–334
Satya yuga 222–223
Satyam 281
Śauklya 119
Shashankāsana 325
Siddhānta 345
Siddhapīṭha 304
Śilpa 239
Śira 239
Śiśira 209–210, 213, 217
Śīta 109, 117, 119, 210–211
Śiva 179, 229–230, 247, 254, 265, 288–289, 292, 294–295, 303–304, 306, 311, 378
Sloka 179, 187–188, 203
Smṛti 223
Sneha 114, 119
Śrī cakra 261, 305, 307, 312
Śrī vidyā 37, 236
Śrīmad bhāgavata purāna 313–314
Śṛṅgāra 81
Śruti 223
Sthairya 119
Sthūla śarīra 46, 54, 107, 242
Strī-graha 177
Suhagans 81–82
Śukla pratipadā 177
Śukra 108, 123, 136, 318, 355–356
Sūkṣma śarīra 46, 49, 51, 53–54, 107, 242–243
Sumbha 307
Suśruta 49, 53–57, 65, 78, 97, 106, 108–109, 118, 123, 132, 209, 217, 356, 359, 364, 371
Susrutas ayurvedas 57
Suṣumṇa 179
Sutras 321, 347
Svadhiṣṭhāna 243, 247–248, 272–275, 278, 280–281, 300, 373–374

Svadhiṣṭhāna 243, 247–248, 272–275, 278, 280–281, 300, 373–374
Svadhiṣṭhāna cakra 247–248, 272–274, 281, 300, 373–374
Svāhā 280–281
Svarāt 224
Svayam-vyakta 241

T

Tākṣaśila 60
Tālu 275
Tamas 319–321, 333–334
Tambulam 81
Tantra 17, 32, 94, 217, 222–227, 230, 232, 234, 272, 304–305, 311–312, 317, 332
Tantrī 229
Tantrik sādhana 224
Tantriks 310
Tapah 280–281, 341
Tāra 289
Tārā 231
Tarka 343, 345
Tarka śāstra 343
Thriputh-aarattu 262–264, 268
Tīkṣṇa 114, 212
Tikta 95, 210, 367, 370
Tretā yuga 222–223
Tridoṣa 50, 53, 55–56, 59, 95, 109, 346
Triphala 57
Tripurasundari 231, 307
Tryaṇuka 50, 350
Tryasarenu 346
Tulasī 43

U

Udāna 245, 335, 360, 376–377
Umānanda 34, 289, 292–296, 375
Unmeṣa 230
Upacaya 188–189, 191–192, 194–195, 199
Upacaya 188–189, 191–192, 194–195, 199
Upacaya sthāna 188, 194–195
Upamāna 49, 343–344
Upanishad 101
Upapīṭha 304
Upāsak 228–229
Upāsana 228–229, 312
Urad 78, 88, 95–97
Ūru 239
Uṣṇa 114, 117, 211
Uttara āṣāḍha 194
Uttarāyaṇa 180, 209, 291
Uttarāyaṇa 180, 209, 291

V

Vāda 345
Vairāgya 179, 249, 295, 338

Vaiśadya 109
Vaiśeṣika 48–50, 64, 331, 343, 346–350, 352
Vaiśeṣika darśana 348
Vaishnavi 307
Vajrāsana 325
Valliyamkavu 33
Varṣā 209, 211, 213, 217
Vasanta 209–210, 213, 217
Vāstu puruṣa maṇḍala 239
Vastu purusha 240
Vāta 50, 56, 59, 97–98, 107, 109–114, 119, 121–122, 124–125, 127, 129, 132, 151–158, 160–162, 164–166, 171, 205, 210–214, 244–246, 291, 360, 369–370
Vāta 95–97, 119
Vāta doṣa 109–112, 132, 151–153, 156, 160, 162, 164, 205, 211–212, 244–245, 291, 360
Vāta doṣa 109–112, 132, 151–153, 156, 160, 162, 164, 205, 211–212, 244–245, 291, 360
Vāta prakopa 111–113, 165
Vāyu 50, 95, 109, 118, 156, 164, 210–211, 244–250, 268, 272, 291, 325–327, 332, 349, 357, 360–362, 365–367, 374–376
Vāyu 50, 95, 109, 118, 156, 164, 210–211, 244–250, 268, 272, 291, 325–327, 332, 349, 357, 360–362, 365–367, 374–376
Vedas 17, 48, 64, 223, 231–232
Venkataramanana binkada rani 228
Vikṛti 122
Visarga kāla 209
Visnupīṭha 304
Visra gandha 114
Viśuddhi 272, 274, 278, 281, 301–303, 308, 376–377
Viśuddhi cakra 272, 274, 301, 303, 308, 376–377
Viśuddhi cakra 272, 274, 301, 303, 308, 376–377
Vitaṇḍā 345
Vīthī 304
Vṛṣabha 192, 196–198, 200, 203
Vṛścika rāśi 192
Vyāhṛti 276, 280
Vyāhṛtis 276, 280–281
Vyāna 245, 335, 360–361, 376

Y

Yōg 32–33, 37, 45–46, 48–49, 138, 157, 186, 224, 259, 319, 325, 331, 337–342
Yōg sūtras 37, 340
Yōga 64, 250, 321, 325, 327
Yōgi 49, 340–341
Yōni 287–289, 300, 305–307, 309–311
Yukti 49, 333

CPSIA information can be obtained
at www.ICGtesting.com
Printed in the USA
LVHW111507260121
677545LV00031B/507

9 781649 198662